"Bles

Destroying The Myth

Many people are sick and dying because of their
unhealthy eating habits and sedentary lifestyles

**It is unsafe to just assume that you can continue to
bless and eat anything and everything you want.
Life and death are set before you as you say grace.
Choose life so both you and your seed may live.**

This is not a Diet, but a Lifestyle!

Jonathan Finley

Faith Publishing Group, Inc.

Contents

Healing • Weight Loss • Cleansing • Detox

Disclaimer

The information provided in this book is offered as an educational and reference volume only. It is not intended to take the place of medical advice from your physician. If you are currently under the care of a doctor, it is advised that you consult your doctor before implementing any of the programs mentioned in this book. "Bless It & Eat It" Destroying the Myth is intended to be used as a preventative tool in addressing many of the afflictions plaguing our society today. This book is intended to help motivate you into making a conscious decision to eat healthier and make exercise a part of your daily routine. Any information acted upon in this book you commence at your own risk

*The author, bookstores, publishers, and distributors present this information for **educational purposes only**. I will not be making any attempt to prescribe a diagnosis or medical treatment. The information in this book is only my opinion, and is based on personal experience and biblical references. If making this change seems too difficult for you, then at least do it for the sake of your children and your loved ones. This is not a diet, but a lifestyle.*

Jonathan Finley

Sickness and disease affects every race and religion on the face of the earth. In a recent study released by the International Society for the Study of Obesity, it stated that obesity and diabetes affects 300 million people worldwide, and that this twin epidemic is expected to shorten life expectancy around the world. The more body weight you carry around, the shorter time you'll likely have to carry it. Thirteen percent (13%) of our population was overweight in 1980. Today, 70% are overweight and 35% are clinically obese. Authorities now agree the average American diet no longer provides the needed nutrition for a foundation of good health. In 2004, the government restructured the food pyramid, putting more fruits and vegetables at the top, replacing meat and dairy groups. Forty percent (40%) of middle class American children are malnourished, and adults fare far worst: upwards to 90%. The number one complaint of corporate America is healthcare costs and the loss of production due to employee sicknesses. The cost of treating just heart disease alone is a staggering $350 billion annually. Many employers can't give more to their employees in the area of bonuses and other incentives, because rising healthcare costs are eating away at their profits.

Christ dying on the cross made no physical changes to our bodies or the animals. All the praying in the world will not remove the fat, cholesterol, and toxins from the food we eat. My friend, God will not miraculously appear and stop you from eating that third hamburger, that fifth piece of chicken, or that second piece of four-layer chocolate cake, mind you all in the same meal. Saying grace and giving thanks is great, but you must give thanks for foods that were meant to be eaten or you will pay the consequences for your decisions. If you sow unhealthy eating habits, you will reap a life of sickness and disease. Stop blessing foods that don't bless you. The Bible starts with nutrition in Genesis, Chapter One, and ends with nutrition in Revelation, Chapter Twenty-Two. The medical and scientific communities all agree that eating more fruits, vegetables, exercising, and reducing the intake of meats, dairy, processed foods and a smoke-free lifestyle can help prevent up to 75% of the afflictions plaguing our society today. Stop, take a moment and ask yourself, "does it really make sense to thank God for foods which have been stripped of all vitamins, minerals, nutrients, and then polluted with a plethora of artificial additives, synthetic vitamins, chemicals, food colorings and preservatives."

I bring you this information with conviction and a clear conscience. I have been practicing this lifestyle for over 25 years. I remember being teased when I was younger because I used fruit juice in my corn flakes instead of milk. Everyone called me seed boy, bird man, and always made fun of what I ate. At every family gathering, the topic was, "let's see what John is going to eat." I really don't know why I stopped drinking milk and started using fruit juices at such an early age. I can only believe that God was cleaning me up in preparation for this predestined assignment.

You see, I have a deep love and passion for children and I see so many of them practicing the unhealthy generational habits of their parents. If something doesn't get our attention soon, our children will never grow up to experience full and productive lives. They will inherit the same illnesses that we pass along to them from our bad eating habits. The predestined plan that God has for their lives will never come to fruition. The enemy will cripple and destroy them from birth to the grave. For example, doctors are now warning that 4 to 6 year old obese children who develop Type 2 diabetes by the age of 14 to 16, raising their possibility of developing devastating complications by the age of 30. They may also suffer with high blood pressure, stroke, kidney failure, cancer, heart disease, and even premature death.

Dry land signifies a new beginning with God. Genesis 1:3 states that, "God gathered the waters below the sky into one place and dry land appeared." Genesis 2:5, "God created man from the dust of the earth," again dry land. Genesis 8:14-15, "by the 27th day of the first month the earth was completely dry. Then God said to Noah, come out the ark." Exodus 14:22, "and the Israelites went through the sea on dry ground." Joshua 3:17, "The priest who carried the ark of the covenant of the Lord, stood firm on dry ground in the middle of the Jordan, while all of Israel passed by until the whole nation had completed the crossing on dry ground." 2 Kings 2:8, "Elijah and Elisha crossed the Jordan on dry land before Elijah went up into heaven in a whirlwind." Jonah 2:10, "So the Lord spoke to the fish and it vomited Jonah onto dry land." In each of these instances, the old experience was being replaced with a new one. I want you to forget about all of your unhealthy generational eating habits, and ask God to help you make a conscious decision to start over dry. When drug addicts go into rehabilitation, part of their treatment involves a drying out process

God has magnificently created us so that by starting over the right way, our bodies can heal themselves. We can have new bones, heart, lungs, liver, and other organs in just one year and, in fact, every seven years, the body will completely regenerate itself if properly nourished. The operative words here are "if properly nourished." Come on! Isn't it worth it for the sake of your health, your children and your loved ones? It's time to make the right choices and become educated with the information you will need to win the battle for your health. Don't just sit back and become another statistic. Be proactive about the health and welfare of your family. We're not just talking about the quantity of years, but the quality of life and good health during these years. We should look forward to the health and vitality experienced by Moses. The Bible teaches us that upon his death at the age of 120, he was yet full of vigor and his eyes had not dimmed. You may think this is impossible, but nothing is impossible with God, as long as we listen, follow, and obey His commands.

Introduction

It has been my misfortune to see both my parents pass away in my lifetime. I watched my father suffer a massive stroke at the age of 47, when I was only 13. This stroke left him speechless and paralyzed for the next 23 years of his life, until he passed away at the age of 70. I always thought I would live to see my mother grow old and grey, and even saw myself one day buying her the dream home she often spoke about. My father taught me how to swim, fish, lift weights, and play ball. I watched one morning in a matter of moments a transformation that will forever be embedded in my memory. One moment he was exercising before heading out to work and the next, he was lying on his back unable to speak or move his body. Just moments earlier he was walking into a bright future. My father had recently been appointed pastor, and had also received a promotion on his job as a medical technician. As I crouched over him, he stared at me in bewilderment as if his entire universe had just stopped. As I looked into his eyes, I painfully realized the fact that our lives would never be the same. I was raised to believe, as long as I blessed my food be fore I ate it, I would suffer no bodily harm. Now I know, you can't just bless and eat anything and everything you want.

Today, so many people are afflicted and dying prematurely as a result of their unhealthy eating habits. It is shocking the number of people who are walking around with acute illnesses, not having the slightest idea of just how close they are to death. Heart disease is the number one killer in the United States, Canada, and Western Europe. Heart disease in the U.S. kills more Americans than the next seven causes of death combined, including cancer, although a third of the deaths could be prevented if people followed better diets and exercised more, according to the American Heart Association.

It goes on to state that nearly 62 million Americans have some form of cardiovascular disease, and nearly a million die from such conditions each year. Every 33 seconds someone dies from heart disease, which accounts for 40% of the deaths annually. What's most surprising, is that heart disease and stroke numbers are not going down and in fact, we are seeing an increase in some groups such as African American women. Since 1984, more women have died each year from heart disease than men. Every minute, a woman dies of a heart attack in this country, and every 13 minutes one dies of breast cancer. Prostate cancer is killing men so fast it is actually frightening doctors. As one doctor stated, "men are dying so fast they're dropping like flies, before ever reaching the age where prostate cancer should be an issue." As you are reading this page, 40 million Americans are walking around with some form of kidney failure and don't even know it. I know of parents who have 1 and 2-year-old infants that have already started taking insulin before they can barely walk or talk. We watch television commercials with the likes of B.B. King talking with a young teenaged boy as they discuss their diabetes situation. Our children have to monitor their blood sugar levels while attending elementary school. There are news reports about young adults committing suicide after taking anti-depressant drugs. As I stated earlier, the enemy is crippling and destroying our children before they can even begin to fulfill the plan that God has for their lives.

The sad thing is every morning we get up and follow the same old routines and even pass these unhealthy habits along to our children. From the time we wake up until the time we go to bed, we do nothing to improve the quality of our health. All of a sudden there's a sharp pain in your chest, and you immediately rush to your doctor for a prognosis. If you are not too late, evasive actions are taken and you are put on medication for the rest of your life. I'm sorry, but God did not intend for us to live this way. It states in Luke 1:53 "He has filled the hungry with good things." Hosea 4:6 says "my people are destroyed because of lack of knowledge." Many people just don't know how to prepare their foods, in what order their foods should be eaten, or what they should and shouldn't eat. So everyday, they subject their bodies to intolerable toxins, parasites, and poisons. The body has no way of coping with these things. After so many years of this, the human body becomes too ravaged and weakened to fight back, and death finally consumes every area of the body.

If you haven't noticed, the majority of people in this country are not born with cancer, heart disease, diabetes, or cataracts. However, an alarming number of them are suffering and dying prematurely from such diseases. It is amazing to think that the human body is comprised of trillions of living cells, yet everything we eat is dead. Listen carefully, *"Death Cannot Feed You Life!"* Again, I will repeat that life saving statement, *"Death Cannot Feed You Life!"* Even the earth is nourished and cleansed on a consistent basis through nature. We have trillions of living cells that require living minerals and nutrients to reproduce. What do you think is happening when we deprive our bodies of living nutrients and minerals that actually bathe and cleanse every cell in our bodies. If Jesus himself instructed us to eat the living bread and drink the living water to survive spiritually, so it is the same physically. It is imperative that we nourish our bodies with living nutrients and minerals. Stop blessing and eating foods that don't bless you!

"Bless It & Eat It" is not some new diet plan or nutritional fad. There are enough of those to go around, and yet we are still in a health crisis. It is not some quick fix or temporary solution. You will not physically live forever by changing the way you eat, because God didn't allow mankind to eat from the tree of life. The information contained in "Bless It & Eat It" has been around since the creation of mankind. It goes behind the scenes and deals with the psychological side of the equation first. It attempts to expose where the real battle for your health starts and who is behind the attack. You can overcome this attack with the five steps to healing program:1) kicking the sugar habit; 2) losing weight permanently; 3) enhancing mood and sleeping better; 4) increasing your energy level; and 5) increasing your odds of not developing diabetes, heart disease, certain types of cancer, obesity, and hypertension. It is amazing to me that our country, with access to the best medical and educational facilities at its disposal, has generation after generation unaware of how to properly nourish their bodies.

"Bless It & Eat It" attempts to explore unhealthy generational foods and the bad habits we practice. Foods such as meat and seafood, are loaded with fat, cholesterol, uric acid, and toxins. White sugar is more destructive and damaging than any other poison, drug, or narcotic, and is an addictive unnatural substance not found in nature. Table salt is pure sodium chloride and is horrific and damaging once it enters the body. White flour has been linked to a host of allergic reactions, and fried foods. There are other unhealthy habits like drinking soda, milk, coffee, smoking, and lack of exercise. These unhealthy generational habits are the culprits behind so many of the medical maladies affecting our society today. It goes to the heart as to why so many of us struggle to overcome our unhealthy eating habits. How the fast food industry over the years has super sized our meals, and now the apparel industry is stretching and super sizing our clothing.

It is easy to recognize that one of the greatest sins in the United States is gluttony. Food has become the god of millions. Many sicknesses that are plaguing mankind stem directly from unhealthy eating habits. Phillippines 3:19 says "whose end is destruction, whose God is their belly, and whose glory is their shame, who mind earthly things." Many of us are praying and waiting for miracles that will never happen until we take the first step and change our unhealthy generational habits. Notice when God delivered the Israelites out of Egypt, the first thing He did was to change their diet. Exodus 16:4 says, "Behold I will reign bread from heaven for you." There is an interesting story in the Bible about a king who had been sickened with a cancerous boil, and was told by the prophet of God that he was going to die. Notice when God allowed this king to live, he was not miraculously healed of his sickness. Instead, God gave instructions through the prophet to have the king's servant place a poultice of figs on the boil. Isaiah 38:21 "Isaiah had said, prepare a poultice of figs and apply it to the boil and he will recover." In the Old Testament, we read how Elisha healed undrinkable water by using salt. 2nd Kings 2:21, "Then he went out to the source of the water, and cast in the salt there, and said, "Thus says the Lord: I have healed this water, from it there shall be no more death or bareness."

In the book of Genesis, we read that Adam and Eve used fig leaves for clothing. It's probably safe to assume that figs were a part of their normal diet. David revived an Egyptian soldier by giving him figs to eat, and Jesus wanted figs when he became hungry. Ironically, Japanese scientist have treated cancer patients with an anti-cancer chemical found in figs. Of 55 patients tested, 7 went into complete remission and 29 into partial remission. Of all fruits, figs contain the highest concentration of minerals. Figs are very rich in potassium which helps to regulate the release of sodium into the blood. Real unrefined Celtic Sea Salt is vitally important for those suffering with heart disease, diabetes, and a host of other illnesses. Figs, in conjunction with Celtic Sea salt, are powerful medicine for those suffering with hypertension, because both are very helpful in balancing and maintaining blood pressure.

C H A P T E R   1

I Thought I was too Young

"I have set before you life and death, blessing and cursing: therefore choose life, that both thou and thy seed may live:" (Deuteronomy 30:19)

The symptoms started out very early in life for me. I wasn't old enough to drink, smoke, or do drugs. I didn't have a job, wasn't married, didn't have any children or bills to pay. I was just basically living what I considered a totally stress-free life. I was young and still in grade school, yet I was always suffering with one illness after another. I had constant migraine headaches, elevated blood pressure, acne, colds, congestion, and chronic fatigue. Because I worked out regularly, I thought I was pretty healthy. Yet, I was so devastated with chronic fatigue that I once thought I had the AIDS virus. So I went to several specialists for medical help, and after numerous tests (including one for the HIV virus which turned out to be negative), I was told there was nothing that could be done for me. Afterwards, I was sent home in the same condition in which I arrived. What was really shocking was the fact that these doctors were equipped with the latest advancements in medical technology. I wasn't living in a third-world country, but in the United States Of America. Still, they had no clue as to what was causing my condition.

After several more years of suffering with chronic fatigue, migraine headaches, and depression, I finally found out on my own what was causing my debilitating condition. I noticed that once I removed refined sugar completely from my diet, I no longer suffered with chronic fatigue, depression, or migraine headaches. Instead, I gained energy, vibrancy, vigor, and all the symptoms I suffered before were completely gone. No longer did I wake up to eat breakfast and immediately start feeling sluggish, sleepy, and lightly depressed. I couldn't believe that something as simple as sugar was causing these severe adverse conditions. No medicine, no therapy, no counseling, just the simple removal of one food group from my diet. Yes, I called sugar "food", but really it is nothing but a chemical drug that is highly addictive and habit forming, similar in form to heroin. As a matter of fact, they both produce the same symptoms, a quick high, and then a debilitating crash. However, I had not yet made the connection between diet and health. You see, for so many years I was told by doctors, family members, and friends, that food had nothing to do with my health. You've probably heard the same information most of your life. I suffered with severe acne to the point where I once stayed out of school for a whole month. I was treated by some of the best dermatologists in Beverly Hills, yet I was told the same thing over and over again...basically that food had nothing to do with my problem. I was just going through adolescence, and the disfiguring of my face by acne was just a part of life. Again I changed my eating habits and started doing some internal cleansing and just like that, my acne problems disappeared.

I was shocked to learn that what I ate could cause so much havoc on my body. From that point on, I started connecting diet with illnesses and realized that what I ate had everything to do with how I looked and felt. Almost twenty-five years have passed since those painful days, and I haven't suffered with any of those illnesses since I made the connection and changed my eating habits. Today, so many people are suffering with illnesses because like I was, they are unaware of the health hazards eating unhealthy foods can cause. I use to always ask myself this question, "If I wasn't born with these conditions, then why do I suffer with them now?" I have been investigating and experimenting with health and nutrition for over 25 years and I am convinced that *you are what you eat*!

To prove this point even further, I once took my family on a vacation to Florida for a week. While in Florida, we went to a friend's house for dinner. Most of the food they served I couldn't eat because of my nutritional lifestyle, but the corn chips they served as an appetizer looked pretty healthy and innocent. After all it was nothing more than just corn, oil, and salt. So I indulged into a food which I hadn't eaten in over 25 years and before long, I was hooked. I ate corn chip after corn chip everyday until the end of my vacation. When the vacation was over, something amazing happened to me. I began breaking out with hives and whelps all over my body, and started itching uncontrollably. My wife thought I had rubbed against some poison ivy while jogging in Florida. I was sure that wasn't the case, and in the back of my mind, I suspiciously knew the culprit was really the corn chips. So I stopped eating them, and started an aggressive detox program along with lots of lemon water and exercise. In just a matter of a few days, all the itching stopped and the swelling began to subside. By the end of week, I had completely recovered and had no other symptoms since.

Because of my nutritional habits and low levels of toxicity within my body, the corn chips had an immediate adverse effect on my health. My body immediately rejected the toxins produced from the ingredients in the corn chips. The hives and itching were a warning to me that my body's pH (potential hydrogen: I'll explain this later) had gone from alkaline to acidic, and was totally out of balance. This imbalance set the wheels in motion and my immune system went to work to flush this poison out of my body. Once I became aware of the situation through the physical manifestations, I had a choice to make. I could continue eating the corn chips and suffer, or discipline my taste buds and save my mental and physical health. You see, not only was I suffering with hives and uncontrollable itching, but it became physically unattractive and emotionally embarrassing. For me, it wasn't a choice at all. My health was more important than a $3.00 bag of Frito Lay corn chips. The chips only cost $3.00 per bag, but the cost to treat the devastating side affects would have cost hundreds of dollars over time. Deuteronomy 30:19 says, "I have set before you life and death, blessing and cursing: therefore choose life, that both thou and thy seed may live:" Why do so many people choose death over life, sickness over health, suffering over wellness?

It seems we are creatures of habit and would rather put our trust in everyone and everything else except God. It would make sense that since God made our bodies, He would know exactly what we should feed it. You see, society tells us how we should look and feel, and what we should eat. When it comes to what we actually should eat, the American diet is nutritiously deficient. If your diet is deficient, then your health is deficient, and this is where the bulk of our health problems start. Everything we eat has been altered and modified from its original nutritional state through industrial proces-sing. We work very hard to earn a living, and we then take our hard-earned money to buy foods that send us into poor health or a prema-ture grave.

The average American is walking around in poor health and doesn't know how close they are to death. A good example of this is my little brother, who at the young age of 34, suffered from congestive heart failure and many other life-threatening complica-tions. Here was a young man in the prime of his life, yet he was totally unaware of the hidden dangers lurking inside his body. He was just a few breaths away from death and a life of medication and rehabilitation. When I got the call, I could not believe the news. My little brother, who was built like Arnold Schwarzenegger and was as strong as an ox, was brought to his knees in a matter of moments by something a million times smaller than him. When we finally got a chance to talk, my first question was concerning the types of food he had been eating. After examining the contents of his diet, I needed no further explanations as to what caused his almost fatal episode.

The following breakdown is just one example of a routine meal. Now you must keep in mind, this was just one meal out of many others in the same day. On any given day, he would eat two packages of Ball Park Frank hot dogs loaded with cheese and other condiments. Then he would top it off with a milk shake and other goodies. This meal was considered normal, and was just one of many in the same day. This breakdown will reveal the outrageously stag-gering amount of fat, cholesterol, and sodium contained in this one meal. Total fat for the hot dogs and cheese alone was a mind blowing **400** grams. I hope you're holding on to your seat. The cholesterol totals were a whopping **1,040** milligrams. Last but not least was the sodium, which totaled an unbelievable **15,500** milligrams. The daily recommended amounts for each of these is no more than **65 grams** of fat, **300 milligrams** of cholesterol, and only **2,400 milligrams** of sodium per day. I purposely left out the bread, harmful chemicals, ar-tificial food coloring, additives, nitrates, preservatives, the pituitary hormones, steroid hormones, thyroid and parathyroid hormones, so-dium ethrobate, gastrointestinal peptides, growth factors, growth inhi-bitors, allergenic proteins, blood, pus, antibiotics, bacteria and para-sites all contained in the meat and dairy. These extra ingredients don't just simply disappear because the food has been cooked; they hang around.

As you can see, this one meal blew the daily recommended guidelines way off the charts. You're probably asking yourself "who would eat this way"? Right! Believe it or not, millions of people over-eat. When was the last time you ate just one serving of anything? No one eats just one serving, because none of us think about serving sizes while we're enjoying the taste and savoring the flavor of our food. Just look on the streets and every elementary, junior high, high school, and college campus around the country. Two thirds of this nation are overweight and a larger number are becoming obese.

There are many diet products, weight loss centers, books, tapes and videos out there, yet people are continuing to grow oversized. The problem is so severe that the federal government has finally stepped in to try and fix this epidemic. This is not a government problem; this is all about making the right choices and having self discipline regarding what you eat. Millions of oversized waistlines are walking around right now without nutritional discipline. In my honest opinion, the serving size information should be removed from all products, and be replaced with warning labels regarding the dangers of overindulgence.

Now it took some time to go out and buy the hot dogs, cheese, and soda. It took time to cook them, eat them, and then wash all of it down with a poisonous soft drink. This was definitely a matter of choice, and not of force. I know right about now you are wondering, "Is he still alive?" The answer is yes, but not without debilitating and disfiguring consequences. You see, one day his heart suddenly stopped beating, and this was the day that his body simply shutdown and said "No More!" The high amount of fat and cholesterol in this meal was clogging his arteries and greatly restricting the flow of blood through out his entire body. The high level of sodium sent his body into toxic shock, which inadvertently set the body into survival mode.

More than 80 trillion cells used the excess water in his body to entomb themselves like a cocoon preventing toxic contamination. This meal caused his body to shift from a healthy alkaline condition to a life-threatening acidic one. His cells were being starved of vital oxygen, vitamins, minerals, and nutrients. They were unable to communicate while in this extended state of survival. They couldn't be cleansed of the deadly toxic waste material building up within this dangerous environment. Blood flow was impeded with the heavy buildup of plaque and fat now clogging the inside of his arterial walls while, at the same time, over 80 trillion oversized cells were trying to travel through the veins in his body. His heart was forced to work harder which caused his entire cardiovascular system to weaken.

Remember, over 80 trillion cells are still starving for oxygen, trying to receive nutrients, trying to excrete toxic waste, and give and receive instructions. With all communication bogged down, cells that were once healthy start degenerating into unhealthy ones. These cells are deformed and cannot help the body correct its' imbalances. The fat and cholesterol began sticking to his artery walls where scar tissue had already developed. Blood clots started forming as this scar tissue was ripped from the artery walls by pressure caused as blood, was being forced to travel throughout his body. These clots are clumps of plaque, cholesterol, fat, and scar tissue that more than 80 trillion unusually enlarged cells now have to maneuver around.

Imagine driving on Interstate 40 West on a stretch of highway that is only two lanes wide. You are smoothly coasting on cruise control at 65 miles per hour. All of a sudden you have to start maneuvering around thousands of trucks and stalled cars scattered on the highway. As your path and rate of speed are hindered, a major accident involving several vehicles happens a couple of miles ahead of you. Now all traffic has come to a complete stop, but to your surprise in your rearview mirror, you notice a speeding freight train coming at you tossing cars in every direction. You're blocked in with no way to escape, so you prepare for the impact of the speeding train. In this scenario, the car you're stuck in is actually your heart which sits in a confined compartment within your chest. All the other vehicles around you are the trillions of cells traveling to their predetermined destinations. The speeding freight train you see looming at you in your review mirror is actually an enlarged blood clot that has become dislodged. The ensuing impact, I'll leave to your imagination.

Eventually, just like a snowball rolling down a steep hill, the clots get larger and larger until arteries become blocked. One day without warning, the clots break away and travel to the heart or to the brain, where they can lead to heart attack or stroke. My younger brother stopped breathing and passed out that day without warning.

Fortunately for him, he was at work and medical help was immediately dispatched to resuscitate him. What would have been the outcome had he been alone and unable to get medical attention? What other unknown conditions are yet lurking behind the scenes waiting for their day? After surviving this ordeal my younger brother was placed on cholesterol, blood pressure, blood thinning, and other medications. These prescription drugs with their toxic side affects made him feel miserable, groggy, and not like himself most of the time.

He suffered from severe swelling in his legs which was also disfiguring and very painful. He lived with the constant risk of suffering a heart attack due to the blood clots in his legs becoming dislodged and traveling to his heart. The circulation to certain parts of his right leg had all but completely stopped. As a result, the skin in this area died and became totally discolored. The swelling and chronic pain in his leg was so severe that he could no longer go jogging or workout. This horrible suffering went on for about two years.

We had a discussion about his condition and what could be done to make it better and make him less dependant on medications. He had gained an enormous amount of weight, which is another horrible side affect of taking prescription drugs. What he thought was harmless snacking almost cost him his life. I was able to help him change his entire medical outlook through some drastic dietary changes along with exercise. We started off by changing all his meals to 80% raw fruits, grains, nuts, herbs, vegetables and 20% cooked fish and vegetables. Within a few months he was totally off all medications, had lost 25 to 30 lbs, and was no longer having the severe painful swelling condition with his leg. The discoloring of his leg was gone and his skin texture almost returned back to normal. He flew out to visit me in Virginia and we went jogging together. The miserable symptoms from the medications were no longer a topic of discussion.

What you eat will definitely determine what you are, how you feel, and how long you live. If your body is overloaded with fat, cholesterol, sodium, and God knows what else, the system becomes clogged up and just like the drain in your house when it gets clogged, nothing can pass through. Every area of his body was slowly and insidiously dying. Your brain consumes 30% to 35% of whatever you eat and must receive fresh oxygen and nutrients to survive. Your heart must pump blood throughout your entire body, reaching and nourishing over 80 trillion cells that make you a complete person. Imagine what happens when these cells don't get the nutrients and oxygen they require to function. These starved cells will start starving your organs and your organs will start starving your body. Now just take a moment and think about how you felt the last time you went without food for an extended period of time. Well, now you know just how your cells feel, but the difference is, your cells stay in this starved state of existence for years and even decades. Many of you may not eat two packages of hot dogs with cheese at one setting, so your episode or crisis will take longer to manifest. Eventually, what you have sown into the temple will produce a harvest, and depending on what you planted will determine the quality, good or bad, of your health. As you are reading this book, some 40 million Americans are at risk of kidney failure. That's right. At this moment, 40 million people are at risk and 90% don't know it. Sadly, 65% of their doctors won't even diagnose this condition because they currently haven't developed a standardized way to test for this fatal debilitating disease.

So many of these same people continue to attend church with you every Sunday and sometimes during the week. They are bishops, pastors, apostles, teachers, prophets, preachers, choir members, ushers, Sunday School teachers, praise team members and leaders, cousins, aunts, uncles, fathers, mothers, sisters, brothers, children and grand-children. They think because no symptoms have manifested that they're not in any immediate danger. In fact, many of them are in for a rude awakening, because kidney failure is just as deadly as heart disease and cancer. The problem with kidney failure is that it is all but impossible to reverse once it reaches the advanced end stages.

The waiting list is very long, and some ethnic groups like African Americans, are at a higher risk of donor rejection than others. What's amazing is that kidney failure is the one of the easiest diseases to prevent. I suffered with kidney failure because I removed salt totally from my diet. At the time, I was unaware of the vital role that real mineral salt plays in keeping the kidneys healthy. Once I corrected this deficiency, the problem totally cleared up. I had to make a choice to make the necessary changes to get my kidneys back in shape. I couldn't depend on anyone else. I had to turn to God, and he sent someone my way with the information I needed and it worked.

Hurricane Katrina clearly revealed why one must depend on God and not the government, scientists, doctors, bishops, pastors, medicine, or money. During the hurricane and immediately following the disaster, it was every man for himself. People were dying because they had no way of getting the medicine they needed. We saw a close-up picture of survival of the fittest. A lot of those who suffered really could have made decisions earlier in their lives that would have prevented the onset of their illnesses. Eating unhealthy foods and practicing unhealthy habits affect every aspect of your life, especially when you face a life-threatening situation. The stress you experience during a crisis really exacerbates any underlying sickness or disease you may be suffering from.

We were all created with one set of organs, and none of us carry around any spare replacement parts. God wants you to take care of the temple and the organs that came along with it. If we are really led by the Spirit and are obedient to what the scripture teaches about honoring God with our bodies, we can avoid unnecessary suffering and afflictions. After watching many who suffered during the hurricane because they lacked their medications, it should send a warning to all of us. It has been proven medically and scientifically beyond a shadow of a doubt that diabetes, hypertension, obesity, cancer, and heart disease are all preventable through healthier lifestyle choices. **Remember, God has placed before you life and death, sickness and disease, so choose life, that you and your seed may live.**

C H A P T E R   2

WARNING:
You Must Read this Chapter

"I have set before you life and death, blessing and cursing: therefore choose life, that both thou and thy seed may live:" (Deuteronomy 30:19)

I purposely placed this chapter in the very front of the book just in case you didn't have a chance to read this entire volume. You would at least have the pertinent information needed to survive the constant battle for your health that rages on twenty-four hours a day. This educational material will help save not only your life and health, but that of your precious loved ones. There is a constant ongoing battle for your health that rages on inside and outside of your body twenty-four hours a day. Every second that you are alive from birth to the grave this battle rages on. This battle affects everything and everyone around you, including your family, friends, jobs, finances, personality, and in some cases even where you decide to live. It is an inescapable and never-ending battle for your very life.

The battle outside your body concerns the pollutants released into the air, oceans, and rivers. Power plants and other sources release emissions into the environment in the form of wet and dry pollutants. These emissions are transported by rain and wind, and deposited into our oceans, rivers, and soils. For instance, mercury transforms into methyl mercury in the water and soil. Humans and wildlife are affected primarily by eating fish containing mercury. We see the impact of this with expectant moms who are warned by their doctors to avoid eating too much fish during pregnancy. The high levels of mercury found in certain fish have been linked to impaired motor and cognitive skills in the unborn developing fetus. This is one of many examples of just how serious this battle for your health is. In some developing industrialized countries around the world, air pollution and poor air quality is responsible for almost a million deaths each year. Because of the 100,000 plus environmental contaminants dumped into our atmosphere for more than the past 50 years, our atmospheric oxygen levels have been reduced in some major industrial cities from 23% to under 9.8%. This situation has become a major culprit in creating a breeding ground for microorganism invasions, because oxygen levels above 13.9 percent are a necessity for killing off these disease-causing pathogens.

The unsettling thing is that atmospheric oxygen content under 10.5 percent sets the stage for cancer. In an environment of less than 7%, life will cease to exist. According to the World Health Organization, air pollution is responsible for almost one million deaths per year. They estimate that about 62 percent of these deaths occur in southeast Asia where the air is heavily polluted with industrial contaminants. Currently, the World Health Organization is working with developing countries in establishing strict air quality control regulations. There are many other stages of this outside battle that time will not allow me to digress into.

There is also a battle raging on inside your body as well. This battle wars to take over your vital organs and disable them, causing all kinds of degenerative diseases such as diabetes, heart disease, cancer, hypertension, obesity, and the list goes on. Concerning the outside battle for your health, there really isn't much you can do to prevent it. However, the one that rages on inside of your body can be overcome by the decisions and habits you practice. You must stop leaving the safety of your health to others, and take responsibility for your own welfare. So many people pitifully find everyone and everything else to blame their poor health problems on. They blame family, friends, relatives, and dark unseen spiritual forces in heavenly places. As if they are literally being forced against their own free will to eat a whole box of Hostess Twinkies, or a 12oz. bag of Frito-Lay Doritos at one setting, or a southern-style fried pork chop dinner smothered with gravy.

Then they're forced to wash this garbage down with a poisonous, highly acidic sugary soft drink called soda pop. By the way, what is so soft about a drink that is so toxic to the body that it requires 32 glasses, that's right 256 ounces of water, just to neutralize one 12-ounce serving. What is so soft about a drink that shuts your entire immune system down for several days. What's so soft about a drink that weakens your bones, teeth, eyes, joints, destroys minerals, feeds cancer, is linked to obesity, diabetes, high cholesterol, kidney failure, and over 120 other diseases. I want to remind you of <u>Deuteronomy 30:19, "I have set before you life and death, blessing and cursing: therefore choose life, that both thou and thy seed may live:"</u> This scripture plainly states that God himself has placed before us life and death, blessings and curses. Not the devil, not our family, friends, co-workers, or any other unseen dark spiritual forces. God himself, has placed in front of each us the choice between life and death. In the Garden of Eden, Adam and his wife were given a choice between life and death in regards to the two trees planted there. The tree of good and evil, and the tree of life. We read that God made Adam and his wife in His image and likeness without the knowledge of knowing good (safety) or evil (danger). In other words, unlike the animals who were created with their own built-in independent internal instinct to judge between good (safety) and evil (danger), man was created to totally depend on God.

In the resent tsunami that struck the shores of Africa, Asia, and India, scientists made a surprising discovery. Many of the animals on the islands hadn't drowned, but instead retreated inland to safety hours before the tsunami struck. However, home video footage showed people wandering out into the surf collecting sea shells, perplexed by the unusual retreat of the waves. We saw footage of people continuing to sunbathe and have fun on the beach, hanging around in their hotels, totally unaware of the impending evil (danger) headed their way.

How was it that the animals knew to start retreating so early into the disaster. They surely didn't receive advance information or evacuation orders from any form of human government. No human corralled them together and led them inland away from the impending evil (danger). The fact is, they didn't need any human warning because their own God-given independent internal instincts kicked in and they knew evil (danger) was headed their way. I've personally experienced many earthquakes while growing up in Southern California. I noticed that often times moments before the earthquakes, the neighborhood dogs would all start barking, as if they could sense something was about to happen. Then all at once they would stop, and the earthquake would immediately follow. Their independent internal instincts still work today. On the flip side, humans with all of their advanced technology, education, and knowledge, were totally oblivious as to the magnitude of the tsunami headed their way.

This incident proves that mankind totally needs to depend on God for his safety and well being, to discern between good (safety) and evil (danger). They should not depend on somebody watching a computer screen or writing some new book about their personal hypothesis regarding what might happen if all the "ifs" line up. It seems the next time we notice the animals running for the jungles, we ought to follow them. This is one reason why God first created man and woman as one person occupying the same body, so that when the time came, God could reveal to mankind that only He could separate them. In this manner, He could forever remind mankind of their requirement to solely depend upon God for all of their needs and well-being. Notice how God brought all the animals to Adam to be named. The animals were brought to Adam each occupying their own individual bodies, both male and female, unlike Adam and his wife who shared the same body. Immediately after Adam named the animals, in the very next verse we read that God put him to sleep, and performed the first human surgery in the history of mankind by separating the two. This act would forever prove of Gods desire to be involved with every aspect of the life of mankind, including his health and well being. God even put together mankind's diet commanding us to eat herbs and fruits as our primary source of food. It's been almost 6000 years since that first diet and today, scientists are just beginning to unlock the hidden secrets of the powerful healing and life-sustaining nutrients contained in herbs and fruits.

Having a clear understanding of this, we can conclude that Adam and his wife made a conscious decision to choose death over life. They willfully chose to operate independently of God's will for them, which resulted in their spiritual separation, causing them both to die spiritually there in the garden. Thus, they were not permitted to eat from the tree of life, and the battle for the health of mankind has raged on everyday since. Today, we have choices to make in pretty much the same way Adam and his wife did. Life and death are placed in front of us everyday in the form of the food we eat, and the unhealthy choices we make. For example, it has been proven beyond a shadow of a doubt that smoking is dangerous and deadly to a person's health. Even-though images are shown of people affected by smoking, the immeasurable amounts of scientific data that is available, coupled with so many hospital beds across the country filled with people wasting away from smoking-related illnesses, people still make a conscious decision to go and purchase cigarettes everyday as if they are invincible. Smoking-related illnesses kill almost 300,000 people per year. Come on, if you are a smoker, all the cards are stacked against you. Don't defile the temple where the Holy Spirit has to dwell. Your body is not yours; it's simply on loan to you from God.

Food was placed in front of Adam and his wife, and just like them, many of us choose death over life. So many people choose to be unhealthy today simply because of the choices they make. What is even more outrageous is that we expect God to come to our rescue and save us every time our health starts failing us. God is merciful and graceful, but we are warned not to test the Lord God. I want to challenge you to get up and make some changes about the quality of your health. Too many people are inactive when they should be proactive in regards to the state of their health. Who fights in a war without taking some kind of defensive proactive posture. In war, the weak and unprepared are the first to die. In the recent hurricane disaster that hit New Orleans, many people died because they lacked medicine. There were so many victims who suffered with diabetes, heart disease, obesity and hypertension.

All of these degenerative disorders are directly linked to poor nutrition and unhealthy choices made on the part of the victim. Yes, in life, we all will get sick from time to time. No one is immune, but we're not suppose to stay sick forever. Depending on how healthy your internal systems are will greatly affect the severity and longevity of your sickness or if you'll even recover. You are fearfully and wonderfully made to remain healthy and vibrant. Your body was designed to perpetually replenish, rebuild, and repair itself when and wherever defects may occur. In order for your body to do this, it must be supplied with the right building materials. In other words, no one goes out and buys defective building materials to build a new house. They carefully purchase new material that usually comes with a warranty. You have to carefully choose what goes into your body and pro-actively guard against substances that will cause the body harm. God makes no mistakes. He has purposely given you life, so don't be in such a rush to end it. I want to educate you with the right information you'll need to take a proactive posture.

First, I recommend that you save your soda and junk food money and go out and purchase a super cleanser to detoxify all of your major internal organs: your liver, lungs, pancreas, kidneys, and intestines. You may also want to follow this up with a parasitic cleanser. Make sure that when you start using any of the two previously mentioned items, take at least two tablespoons of extra virgin, first cold pressed olive oil sprinkled with a little Celtic Sea Salt as this will help to keep your intestines lubricated and provide extra minerals to aid with detoxing. Also, scientists have reported that in Mediterranean countries, men who use olive oil almost exclusively have virtually no incidents of colon cancer. As your body detoxifies itself, you will automatically start losing weight and notice dramatic increases in your energy level. Now that we've cleansed your intestines of years of toxic build up, pathogens, and parasites, we can help start the healing process that will get you on track to winning the battle for your health. You'll need to start a daily routine of rebuilding and balancing you body's pH, your ratio of good and bad bacteria (intestinal flora), and your immune and endocrine systems.

Everyone born in this country needs to start all over again and reset their body's internal health-saving pH balances. When you were born, you were pumped with all kinds of drugs, antibiotics, and vaccines. Prescription and over-the-counter medications are highly toxic to the body, and antibiotics totally destroy both your good and bad bacteria (intestinal flora). This causes your body to remain unbalanced the majority of your life, setting the stage for chronic diseases and sicknesses to include weight gain, acne, migraine headaches, arthritis, digestive disorders, poor vision, colds, flus, sinus problems, and many other common ailments. These symptoms are just the beginning warning signs of system failures, and if not corrected, lead to more severe degenerative diseases such as diabetes, hypertension, cardiovascular disease, and obesity. Once this imbalance is corrected and maintained, you will no longer have to deal with common illnesses. More importantly, you'll be able to prevent the onset of more severe degenerative complications.

To accomplish this monumental task, you will need to do the following: eat a large, dark green, leafy salad everyday and pile on the cucumbers, tomatoes, broccoli, cauliflower, onions, seeds (like raw almonds, sunflower, pumpkin, and ground flaxseed, etc.) Instead of conventional salad dressings which will totally void any health benefits you could have gotten from the salad, use a mixture of apple cider vinegar, extra virgin olive oil, Celtic Sea Salt, and your choice of herbs. This is probably the most important daily meal of your entire life. The only fluid you should ever drink is distilled water and occasionally your own all-natural fruit drink juiced at home. Never drink liquids with a healthy meal. Notice I said never with a healthy meal unless you're trying to lose weight. In such cases, distilled water is perfectly fine. The juice contained in all of your fruits and vegetables is naturally distilled through nature. Sprinkle Celtic Sea Salt on all of your meals to help aid with digestion. Ensure that all of your starches and proteins are eaten separately. This will help to avoid acid reflux and assist you with losing weight and keeping it off.

For the first three to four weeks, a couple of cloves of garlic should be taken daily to help rebuild and strengthen your immune system and suppress the growth of unhealthy bacteria. Take a teaspoon of apple cider vinegar to help mask the garlic odor that may result. Some blood purification also may be needed in the form of grapefruit seed extract or grape seed extract. The use of the powerful herbal sweetener stevia will help promote the growth of healthy bacteria and has other great benefits. A powerful combination to help replace the good bacteria would be to combine stevia with raw organic unsweetened yogurt made from goat's milk if possible or raw organic cow's milk. A daily detox drink of distilled water, ½ fresh lemon, ½ teaspoon of cayenne pepper, and a little stevia will help alkalize your body's pH, boost your energy level, and destroy any polyps that may have developed over the years along your intestinal walls.

Make sure you get out and exercise regularly and enjoy plenty of sunshine. Get a lot of rest by going to bed between the hours of 9 and 10 pm. If these hours are too early, then you should lay down during the day for at least one hour. This will help with proper blood circulation since the heart has to pump harder when you are up on your feet all day, because gravity pulls most of your blood into your legs. Whenever possible, use only herbs to treat whatever ailment pains you. All herbs are alkaline and an alkaline environment promotes healing and overall wellness. Remember, I have included a list of foods and habits you should adopt in **Chapter 6.** I hope you will arm yourself and get into this battle to save your health and that of your precious loved ones. You have the choice between life and death, sickness and health. God wants you to choose life so that both you and your seed may live.

If you are currently suffering from the following, then read on: heart disease, cancer, diabetes, hypertension, obesity, are always tired and have no energy, feeling down, suffering mood swings or bouts with depression, always catching colds, flus, suffering with sinus problems, poor vision, acne, eczema or other skin disorders, having to take antacids after every meal, suffering with irritable bowl syndrome, respiratory conditions, congestive disorders, PMS, hot flashes. If you are suffering from a myriad of other ailments I didn't mention, please stop right now and proceed to **Chapter 12.** This chapter will teach you how to become aggressively proactive in protecting your health.

Ultimately, it is the responsibility of each and every person to do whatever it takes to stay healthy. It is not up to the church, government, friends, family members, or even God himself. I want to impress upon you not to procrastinate and waste time, because time is not on your side. The billions of unhealthy bacteria, parasites, molds, and fungus that are presently living inside your body are not going on vacation. They will continue to rob you of your health and state of well being until you forcefully evict them. They must be immediately evicted through proper internal cleansing and blood purification. The sooner you start, the better you will start feeling. Can you imagine only having to deal with the symptoms of a cold or flu, but never really developing one. Can you imagine living life full of energy, vibrancy, vigor, and free of medications or doctor bills. Can you imagine fewer sick days and time off work, making your employer feel glad they hired you. Can you imagine having people walk up to you on the street or call to ask you what they can do to save their health. You're the light of the world and should shine bright enough for every one to see. Everyone wants the best for themselves and their families. God has given us the very best He has to offer, His all-natural creation. **Remember, God has placed before you life and death, sickness and disease, so choose life, that you and your seed may live.**

CHAPTER 3

Where's the Church and "The Good Shepherd"

"I have set before you life and death, blessing and cursing: therefore choose life, that both thou and thy seed may live:" (Deuteronomy 30:19)

An astronomical $600 billion dollars was spent last year on healthcare costs in this country. I'll repeat that staggering figure for shock value...an unbelievable $600 billion dollars was spent just on healthcare last year. Half of that $600 billion came from believers who are still sick, still seeing doctors, still medicated, and still spending time either bed ridden or in hospitals. We all get sick, but we shouldn't stay medicated and sick our entire lives. A staggering $300 billion dollars was stolen from the Kingdom of God, and millions of believers today are still sick and suffering unnecessarily. Look how well the enemy is advancing against the kingdom by robbing us of our finances, our time, and our health.

What's really baffling is the fact that both the medical and scientific communities have recently stated that almost 75% of these illnesses are all preventable, and are caused by unhealthy eating habits, smoking, and lack of exercise. Satan is full of wisdom and knows that finances, time, and good health are all needed to effectively further the work of God's Kingdom here on earth. It is amazing to me to see the number of sick and suffering people who go to church week after week, month after month, year after year, and decade after decade. Churches all across this country are full of congregations who are taking medications or suffering with some form of sickness. They are taught about how to avoid going to hell, and how important it is to have a close and personal relationship with God. They are taught how to tithe and give their best offering to help the church fund its next mega-project. They are taught how much they are possessed and forced against their own will by some dark spiritual force into a life of helplessness and gluttony.

These poor congregants attend church week after week, are told they must have faith in God, and faith must have works of obedience following it. They are told to just trust in God and everything will work out and if it doesn't work out, somehow it was all a part of God's master plan for their lives. This couldn't be further from the truth. The fact is they have been uneducated, misinformed, and misguided when it comes to nutrition and the temple of God (our bodies). For so many years, the church has expected our secular gover-nment and public educational institutions to teach us about keeping our bodies (God's temple) healthy. How can a government and educational system that doesn't even acknowledge God or the fact that He created mankind, be expected to teach us anything about sound Biblical nutrition. You wouldn't seek guidance from a drug dealer or a thief to discuss your financial retirement plans. So why expect institutions that won't even allow the name of Jesus to be mentioned in public, educate the body of Christ as to how to keep His temple (our bodies) clean and healthy?

Just look at congregations in churches all around this country. People are needlessly suffering and dying and so are their children. Some have physical manifestations such as obesity, hypertension, and diabetes. Others show signs of some sort of mental disorder and are classified by the exorcism department, when in fact, they're constantly starved of vitally important minerals, vitamins, nutrients and are totally out of balance. They are told that suffering may endure for a night, while the parishioner is loading up on toxic medications with warning labels about potentially fatal side affects. The fact that all drugs cause side affects disproves the fact of them being an exact science due to the side affects themselves. Scientist now confirm that although taking an aspirin a day may lower the risk of heart attack, those who take an aspirin a day greatly increase their chances of premature death and suffering due to intestinal bleeding and hemorrhagic stroke. James 1:8 states, "A double minded man is unstable in all of his ways." Either taking aspirin is safe for you or it isn't.

I'll repeat this again, your brain consumes 30% to 35% of whatever you eat. Your brain functions off of electrical impulses enabled by the minerals your supposed to get through proper nutrition.

These minerals are removed from the food supply through industrial processing and mineral-depleted soils, then replaced with toxic chemicals, fertilizers, herbicides, pesticides, and dangerous nitrates, sodium erthrobate, growth hormones, and aluminum silicate, just to name a few. On top of this, we constantly pump our bodies with deadly poisonous sugar, which is nothing more than a chemical drug and is not mentioned once in the entire Bible. Our only other source of naturally available minerals is from real sea salt, which is also stripped and processed by the time it reaches the food supply and our dining room tables. Your brain is now like an eight-cylinder car trying to operate on just two cylinders. All eight cylinders have to operate or your car won't function. Remember I told you earlier that your body is incapable of using and processing synthetic vitamins and minerals added to our foods and sold in vitamin stores. God did not create you out of synthetic material, but real earth-based minerals and water. These minerals, when sold in their commercial state, are sold in dangerously high and unbalanced concentrations.

Your body is made up of natural earth-based minerals and will only recognize and assimilate these types of ingredients. Just look at it this way, your body is comprised of 75% water. It doesn't matter how many synthetically-fortified, thirst-quenching products you drink. Nothing can ever replace the need for natural water. Real minerals enable your cells to communicate effectively and reproduce after their kind. Without the proper resupply of minerals, your body and mind will not be able to function clearly or properly. Just look at the outrageous level of violence and social dysfunction in our society today. People are becoming more and more violent and agitated as they become more toxic. No one can function properly, because 24 hours a day, we are constantly being exposed to polluted air, hormone-injected fast food, chemical-laden processed foods, toxic tap water, dehydrating alcohol, coffee, soda, dangerous prescription drugs, addictive narcotics, poisonous sugar, deadly table salt, violent movies, offensive music, and sexually explicit video games. If you take the batteries out of your flashlight, it will lose the ability to function properly and produce light. If all of the minerals in your brains are removed and replaced with junk, it won't function properly either.

All of our foods today are over processed, overcooked, and totally void of all nutrients and minerals. Making matters even worse is the fact that our foods are loaded with highly toxic refined sugar, which again is not mentioned one time in the entire Bible. Then to add insult to injury, of the 87 minerals and trace minerals that naturally occur in real Celtic Sea Salt, 85 of these minerals are removed through industrial processes and sold to other industries for profit. The only two remaining minerals are sodium and chloride in dangerously high concentrations that we use as table salt, and are dangerously toxic to all humans, animals, and fish. After the salt is processed, it is bleached to make it turn white. Then brain-poisoning aluminum is added along with other anti-caking ingredients to keep it from clumping together, making it flow easily out of the container. Sugar or some other type of sweetener is added to mask the bitter taste of the additives.

Fish from the ocean that are placed in fish tanks where refined table salt is used will die immediately. These fish are born and live in a salty environment all of their lives. Now instead of drinking lots of distilled water and exercising to force this junk out our bodies, we load up on nutritionally-depleted fast foods and soft drinks, making ourselves even more toxic. This extended condition overworks the body and stresses out the organs that are responsible for keeping our bodies cleansed. You can't effectively deal with external outside stresses unless you remove the things causing internal stresses first.

These foods actually leach and destroy the available minerals we have left in our bodies. This condition forces our body to tap into our reserve mineral supply of calcium and magnesium which is stored in our bones, teeth, and joints keeping them strong and healthy. Your body can't function physically or mentally without having all 87 minerals, in the same way our English language becomes useless if just five letters are removed from the alphabet. All 26 letters in the alphabet are needed in order to keep the English language useable and understandable. Without the proper balance of these 87 minerals, you will develop all kinds of symptoms of mineral deprivation. People who are bipolar or manic depressant are given lithium, a trace mineral found in real Celtic Sea Salt, to treat their condition. Why not just leave the lithium in the salt so these mental conditions don't develop? People who suffer with indigestion take Tums, Rolaids, Milk of Magnesia, and Pepto-Bismol which contains magnesium which naturally occurs in real Celtic Sea Salt. Why not just leave these minerals in the salt so people don't suffer indigestion? Too much magnesium in the blood can cause heart, central nervous system, and kidney problems.

Without these minerals in their God-created natural balances, our bodies are unable to remain healthy, and succumb to all kinds of sicknesses, diseases, and mental illnesses. Yes, we are pumping ourselves and our children with poisonous, mineral-robbing refined sugar, which is not mentioned once in the Bible from Genesis to Revelation. Our only true source of non-synthetic minerals is removed through industrial processes for the love of money manipulated by Satan. Real mineral-rich sea salt is mentioned in the Bible 47 times, and was commanded by God to be sprinkled on every sacrifice offered up by the priest as a perpetual covenant of peace.

This was an eternal commandment given to mankind from God as a sign of His promise to be at peace with Him upon forgiveness of his sins. The throne of King David was established by God with a perpetual covenant of salt that included a promise of eternal peace. King David experienced this peace for 40 years while he reigned as Israel's King until his death at age 70, as well as his son King Solomon, until he disobeyed God's will and the kingdom was again divided. This covenant of peace will eventually be fulfilled in Christ when He returns and establishes His eternal Kingdom, and reigns in total peace forever. Today, Celtic Sea Salt has the remarkable ability to restore peace and balance to our whole body, both mentally and physically. It is the only salt where doctors can actually watch as calcium enters the body's bloodstream and travels directly to an injury to start repairing it. With our bodies out of balance, we develop afflictions and are forced to rely on doctor visits and toxic medications for our survival. After the recent disaster shown around the world of people suffering and dying because of lack of medicine following Hurricane Katrina, I hope we all have learned an invaluable lesson: *prevention is the best insurance policy*. Many of these deaths could have been prevented, according to the medical and scientific community, through healthier lifestyle decisions. What happens next time when instead of having to wait five days, it takes two weeks for help to arrive. What if the next time a much larger area is impacted that encompasses more than just the gulf coast states.

Medications come with warning labels, warning you of the

clear and present dangers you face while taking them. Does not the Bible give us warnings about those who indulge in sinful habits. Does it not warn us that those who continue in sin will suffer death. When a person continues in sin, they are simply adding more deadly sinful conditions on top of other deadly sinful conditions. This sinful life-style is poisoning their souls with toxic sinful habits that will eventually lead to death. Sin can't forgive sin, nor can it produce any kind of healing powers, because the Bible warns that the wages of sin is death. Whenever you take medications to treat a sickness, you are adding another toxin on top of the toxic condition that caused you to become sick in the first place. Why do medications cause side affects and come with warnings of potentially fatal complications? The answer is because they are toxic. The body becomes more acidic and oxygen deprived and is unable to produce the internal power it needs to heal itself. This acidic and oxygen-starved environment forces our cells to degenerate, thus reproducing other degenerated cells. These degenerated cells reproduce new degenerated tissues that are unable to help the body repair itself. So we start to develop degenerative diseases such as diabetes, heart disease, cancer, obesity and hypertension.

It is a perpetual condition that we now see being passed on to children from their parents. More and more children are being born with and are starting to develop degenerative diseases, passed down from generation to generation...an assembly line of sick bodies unable to heal themselves. So we have more and more medications, spend more and more money than ever before, and no one is actually being healed. In the same way that sin can't heal sin, medications can't heal sicknesses, because both are toxic and cause more problems than they actually fix. A sinful lifestyle is toxic to our soul, in the same way medications are toxic to our bodies. We treat diabetes with medications that, over time, destroys our kidneys which, in the end, takes our lives, but not without first suffering through painful complications and more medicine.

Let us now examine the average after-church Sunday soul food dinner. This one meal is just as toxic, and causes just as many potentially deadly side affects as medicine and sin. Listen, just because you don't suddenly drop dead doesn't mean that you are not dying. It's the same way that many people sin for several years and don't just abruptly die. In fact, the truth of the matter is they're dying and really are already dead spiritually, because sin has separated them from a life-infusing relationship with God. Let's get back to the after-church Sunday soul food meal. The fried chicken, macaroni and cheese, honey glazed ham, fried fish, candied yams, mashed potatoes and cooked collard greens with fatback. Hey!!! Stop salivating. I know your taste buds are starting to water, but this is just a book, you can't eat it. Where was I. Oh yes. Let's continue with the menu. We have overcooked mixed vegetables, overcooked cabbage with salt pork, smothered pork chops, roast beef, corn bread, corn pudding, peach cobbler, sweet potato pie, bread pudding, four-layered double chocolate cake with whipped chocolate icing, sweet tea, punch, and soda.

This entire meal is loaded with deadly, toxic refined sugar, mineral-depleted poisonous table salt, parasites, pathogens, chemical additives and preservatives, steroids, antibiotics, uric acid, pus, growth hormones, and only God knows what else. After eating this poisonous/toxic and highly acidic meal, a huge dark cloud descends upon you and you can barely walk or move from your seat. It's as if someone has just zapped every ounce of energy from your entire body. You almost drift into a coma as you fight to keep your eyes open. Someone has to find you a brace to keep your neck from breaking, as your head bobs uncontrollably. Your body sinks deep into the couch as your eyelids fight madly to stay open, but to no avail. You are physically unable to fight this dark cloud any longer. You start drifting away until you are forced to fall asleep. Some people often develop headaches after finishing one of these marathon meals. Unbeknownst to you what's really happening is your body is actually trying to save your life since you don't have the discipline to do it yourself.

You see your body functions almost like the gas tank in your car. When you fill your car with gas, your car will only go as far as the full tank will allow. Once the tank becomes empty, your car will roll to a rest and stop operating until you refill it with more gas. The gasoline is your car's source of energy. In the same way, your body receives its supply of energy every night for the next day while you are asleep. Fifty percent of this energy is reserved to keep the body's internal organs functioning: heart, brain, kidneys, lungs, liver, muscles, etc. The rest of the energy is reserved to help aid the stomach with digestion. The problem with this soul food dinner is that it requires a lot of energy to digest, up to 75%-80% more than the body can afford to give up. Because food has been cooked to death, all of its naturally occurring digestion-aiding enzymes have been destroyed. The body now has to use all of its energy just to deal with this problem, so it gives up what it can and then goes into survival mode.

The brain, sensing this threat to the body's energy supply, orders the body to start shutting down in order to save your life. If the brain didn't force you to fall asleep, it would have to steal energy from other organs, thus impairing their ability to function properly. Even the brain itself could be compromised if energy reserves are threatened, so it shuts the body down. The body has a built-in security mechanism that will only give up 50% of its energy supply to aid with digestion and that's it. The rest is held in reserve so you don't kill yourself. That's right. If it wasn't for God's magnanimous grace, you would actually commit suicide while eating. As I stated in **Chapter 4, you are fearfully and wonderfully made.**

A more healthier meal would be one that is energy rich and not contaminated with refined sugar, table salt, and God only knows what else. We are not taught how to properly combine our food to help aid the body with digestion. Instead, we eat our foods improperly combined and grossly overcooked, and then wonder why we're so uncomfortable and tired after each meal. We don't understand why we can't fit into our clothes anymore, and why we are always suffering with some type of affliction. We continue eating these marathon illness-producing meals because no one has educated us. The pastor is also eating this meal, so it must be healthy and highly favored of the Lord. At the same time, you notice that both you and the pastor are starting to develop the same types of ailments. He begins taking medicine for diabetes and hypertension and so do you.

When we don't recover from our ailments or they develop into life-threatening complications, we are simply told that it's all a part of God's master plan for our lives. His great master plan is that you continue going to church week after week, giving your talent, time, and money. Unfortunately, your health continues to deteriorate, along with your children and other family members. Before long, the entire family is suffering with the same illnesses as the pastor, and they are now told they will become hereditary. Yes, it's all a part of God's master plan that you, the pastor, your immediate family, relatives, and yet unborn children will all suffer and be afflicted with degenerative diseases. As you read this section of the book, I'm sure without trying too hard you can think of at least five people suffering with some form of affliction or disease such as diabetes, cancer, heart disease, obesity, hypertension, high cholesterol, acne, constant fatigue, sinus problems, allergies, etc. I told you that you wouldn't have to think too hard. These are your friends and relatives who go to church with you week after week, month after month, and year after year.

It is not a part of God's master plan that you should suffer with these conditions any more than it's any part of His master plan that anyone should go to hell. Hebrews 8:6 says, "But now hath He obtained a more excellent ministry, by how much more He is the mediator of a better covenant, which was established upon better promises." Listen, allergies, colds, acne and headaches are all a form of sickness. Just because you don't look or feel sick, doesn't mean by any stretch of the imagination that you are healthy. If you don't believe me, just go to any hospital or cemetery and you'll see millions of examples of people who thought they were healthy, people who were totally unaware of just how sick they really were until it was too late. Everyday, millions of people are diagnosed with life-threatening illnesses, and are told they only have a few months or few years to live. Without any warning signals or advance symptoms, just out of the blue one day the devastating news comes. These are believers who probably have more faith and are more committed to the church than you are. The problem has nothing to do with their faith or commitment; but everything to do with an unhealthy life-style.

According to the American Heart Association and the American Cancer Society, up to 75% of these afflictions are all totally preventable. So why are we yet continuing to kill ourselves and our loved ones? In all actuality, they were sick and had symptoms long before they ever received the grim news. The body was giving off signs for years. The problem is they were not taught what to watch for. The church has expected us to learn about health from our carnally thinking public education institutions that don't even believe that God created man-kind. They certainly wouldn't teach us that God has put things in the earth to naturally heal our bodies. These schools don't teach anything about moderation or honoring God. As a matter of fact, when your child gets sick, they are taken to the nurse's office where they wait for you to come and pick them up. The nurse doesn't pray with your child or read to them what the Bible teaches about health and wellness. Yet, the church expects the public school system to teach its members how to be healthy. What's amazing is the fact that over all these years of miseducation, and the staggering number of sick people, the church still seems to believe that it is not its responsibility to look out for the health and wellness of its parishioners. The congregation continues to ignore the signs, and believe that they're all just a part of everyday life–every headache, acne breakout, digestive problem, heartburn, skin condition, cold, flu, toothache, joint pain, allergic reaction. All these are small eruptions to what is really brewing deep inside your body.

Almost like a volcano before a major eruption are hundreds and thousands of smaller eruptions. It could be just the exuding steam or small undetectable earthquakes. For years and years, your body will give off small signs because you are so fearfully and wonderfully made, and your body was designed to survive. This is why so many people live with degenerative diseases for years and have no idea how close to death they actually are. As I am writing this book, almost 40 million Americans are in danger of kidney failure and don't even know it. What is more frightening is doctors fail to diagnose almost 65% percent of these cases. Just think, you will visit your doctor many times in your lifetime, and he won't even diagnose you with kidney failure until it becomes a life threatening affliction.

I read an amazing article in the newspaper about a woman who worked as a health department staffer for almost 30 years of her life. She was now suffering with end-stage kidney failure, and was undergoing four-hour sessions of painful dialysis treatments three times a week. The sad news was the fact that she will most likely spend the rest of her life going through this weekly excruciating nightmare. Understand, this problem didn't just happen overnight. She had been battling with high blood pressure since her youth. This eventually led to diabetes, which eventually lead to kidney failure. People with kidney failure have a 25% higher chance of suffering from cardiovascular disease. Look at the domino affect of one sickness after another. I'm sure that every time she went to church and gave her time, talent, and money, she believed God was going to heal her of the high blood pressure, then diabetes, and eventually kidney failure. Right about now, I'm sure some super spiritual person would ignorantly say, "Well maybe she didn't ask God to heal her, or she didn't have enough faith." People with this mentality really get under my skin and should never be asked for advice. While they are encouraging you to just have faith and believe in God, they're running out to the doctor and then home to a medicine cabinet full of prescription drugs.

When Jesus had finished teaching the 5000 and was told by the disciples to send them away hungry, how much faith would it have taken for Him just to simply pray over them and miraculously remove their hunger pains. He had already turned water into wine, could speak to the wind and calm raging storms. He had the ability to raise the dead, walk on water, give sight to the blind, make the mute speak and the deaf hear. He had supernatural powers to speak to unclean spiritual forces and subdue them. He himself would soon be resurrected and ascend into heaven. With all of this power and faith, He could have easily just spoke to them and fulfilled their physical needs with a supernatural non-nutritional miracle.

What I love about Jesus is the fact that he didn't act super spiritual or deeply intellectual, but instead very practical. Even though he had infinite knowledge and wisdom, He never once paraded it. These poor hungry people had given Him their time, talent, and money, and in return, He supplied their physical needs with physical substances. Jesus multiplied two fishes and five loves of bread feeding over 5000 people. On another occasion, he fed 4000 people and even cursed a fig tree, because it could not supply his physical needs. I'm quite sure Jesus had enough faith to pray over Himself.

He called himself "The Good Shepherd" because he never failed to understand the spiritual and physical needs of his sheep. If all we needed were spiritual miracles to survive on, God would have never given us physical food to eat. I'm not knocking prayer or faith because even doctors and scientists will tell you that there is unbelievable healing power in prayer and faith. I pray more than anyone I know, but I also honor God's earthly temple (my physical body)

more than anyone else I know. <u>John 16:17 reads, "Nevertheless I</u>
<u>tell you the truth, it is expedient for you that I go away: for if I go</u>
<u>not away, the comforter will not come to you: but if I depart I will</u>
<u>send Him to you.</u>" Now think about this scripture for a second. Why
would Jesus send the comforter to come and occupy sick people; people who are too sick to do anything for the kingdom of God?

Jesus taught, lived, and led by example. He showed us how
a good shepherd should keep and tend the flock. Pastors and leaders,
if your members see that you're always sick, suffering, and taking
toxic medications to treat what's ailing you, they'll think it's okay for
them also. We can plainly see that scientific findings are based upon
false premises and not true verifiable facts. This is why all synthetic
man-made medications come with labels warning of multiple dangerous and potentially fatal side affects. This, in itself, proves the drugs
are not the exact science they claim, because the side effects nullify
the exact science. Today, many religious establishments and believers
accept and follow the teachings of the scientific and medical
community. Because of this, they live in constant transgression of
almost every fundamental principle of life, that God established when
it comes to nourishing the temple and how we should live here on
earth.

In Genesis 1:29, we are given every herb bearing seed for
food to promote health and longevity, and in Revelation 22:2, it reads
that the leaves shall be for the healing of the nations. Raw seed
bearing leaves without ranch dressings, bacon bits, and fat back, were
a part of man's first diet and will continue to be through out his
eternal existence. Most of us haven't eaten raw leaves our entire lifetime, and according to scripture, they promote healing and well-ness.
The quick-fix solution of drugging and medicating is now what is
causing the disease epidemic in this country. This puts hospitals and
doctors as the number three killer in the country, maiming almost 300
thousand people every year. Satan already has the world exposing us
to as much toxic and acidic junk as possible. We don't need to make
his job any easier, but more difficult.

Don't worry, the medical and pharmaceutical industry won't
go broke and start laying off people because the body of Christ is
healed. They have enough existing and up and coming new customers
to keep them wealthy until Christ returns. Three hundred billion

dollars is a lot of wealth that is being transferred from the church. Satan is very wise, deceitful, and cunning with a whole lot of old tricks and schemes. He understands that some folks love God too much to just outright fornicate or commit adultery. He knows quite well that he cannot force you into sin because of your commitment and sincere love for God. Since he can't force you to commit sin, he cunningly gets on your side. Satan knows that everyone, especially saints, love to eat on Sunday after church. So he attacks the church through what we eat, which affects the overall health and well-being of the temple where the Holy Spirit dwells.

It ultimately affects our ability to effectively minister and reveal the glory of God to other people. We can unknowingly hinder the work of the Spirit if this temple (our bodies) is leaking, damaged, and falling apart. You would find it quite difficult to comfortably live in a house where the roof is damaged and leaking, windows broken out, toilet inoperable, no air, electrical problems, no heat, and the foundation is coming apart. As a matter of fact, you probably wouldn't even consider living in a house in this type of decrepit condition. In the same way, the Holy Spirit would have a hard time using a body that is compromised by sickness and disease and totally falling apart. Corinthians 3:16-17 says, "Know ye not that ye are the temple of God, and that the Spirit of God dwelleth in you. 17. If any-one destroys God's temple, God will destroy him; for God's temple is sacred, and you are that temple. Further we are reminded in chapter 6:19 & 20, "Know ye not that your body is the temple of the Holy Spirit which is in you, which ye have of God, and ye are not your own." 20, "For ye are bought with a price: therefore glorify God with your body, and in your spirit, which are God's."

We are clearly instructed here that our bodies don't belong to us, but to God. He commands that we glorify him with both our body and in our spirit. Today, too many believers in the church are honoring God with their spirit, but totally disregarding Him when it comes to their bodies. When He refers to honoring Himself with our bodies, He's referring to more than just restraining from sexual immorality or praying four hours a day. He's also speaking of not smoking, being drunk with wine, using illicit drugs, gluttony, or knowingly doing anything to defile the temple of God. Anything you put into your body that alters its natural balance defiles the temple of God.

Many people today are unable to effectively do the work of the ministry, because their bodies are broken down and worn out. They neither have the strength, energy, mental alertness, or sound physical health to go out into the highways and hedges and compel others to come to Christ. They're too busy worrying about their own health to try and save someone else. The adverse side affects caused by the medications they take severely impacts their mental and physical wellness. Now by the looks of some believers, they would have a hard time trying to convince anyone to follow them. I mean come on, who would want to follow someone who looks like they can't make it very far themselves? If we were honoring God with our bodies, this would not be the case. The Holy Spirit is gentle, and will not force you to do anything against your will. He is always looking for someone who is willing and able to be used. If you resist long enough and continue to defile the temple, He will be forced to find another temple to operate in. It would go well with you both physically and spiritually if you were to simply honor God with your body and in your spirit. **Remember, God has placed before you life and death, sickness and disease, so choose life, that you and your seed may live.**

C H A P T E R   4

You are Fearfully and Wonderfully Made

"I have set before you life and death, blessing and cursing: therefore choose life, that both thou and thy seed may live:" (Deuteronomy 30:19)

I will praise thee: for I am fearfully and wonderfully made: marvelous are thy works: and this my soul knows very well. For my frame was not hidden from you, when I was made in secret and skillfully wrought in the lower parts of the earth. Your eyes saw my substance being yet unformed. In your book they were all written, the days fashioned for me when as yet there were none of them."(Psalms 139: 14-16). Mankind is essentially made up of the following airborne elements: 96% oxygen, hydrogen, nitrogen, and carbon, which constitutes the breath of life God blew into our nostrils. God then completed the remaining four percent of our makeup from the dust of the ground consisting of potassium, copper, gold, nickel, platinum, silver, aluminum, calcium, iron, titanium, zinc, arsenic, iodine, tin, uranium, mercury, and over 70 other minerals and trace minerals. Genesis 2:7 says, "And the Lord God formed man of the dust of the ground (here we have dry land indicating a new beginning) and breathed into his nostrils the breath of life, and man became a living being.

All forms of human life start out with the union of a male sperm and a female egg. This marriage is consummated within an ocean of mineralized saline fluids while the two remain enclosed within the embryonic sack of the mother's womb. These minerals are the dust of the earth that transform this newly joined couple into an embryo, then a fetus, and eventually a baby, one that ultimately has grown over three billion times in size and weight since its conception. So this earthly temple God created as a residence for man's spirit was built from mineral and atmospheric elements owned by God. These same naturally alkaline mineral elements are vitally important to maintaining a healthy temple free of sickness and disease.

The molecular structure of proteins are analyzed as nitrogen, carbon, oxygen, and hydrogen. Carbohydrates are simply a carbon molecule attached to a water molecule. Vitamins and fats are just a combination of oxygen, carbon, and hydrogen. Signs of sickness and disease are plainly our fearfully and wonderfully created temples responding to the foreign acidic toxic materials we allow to enter them. This is accomplished through what we drink, eat, breathe, and bathe in which, over time, injures and destroys our cells, immune system, and eventually the overall condition of our health.

Scientists have concluded their studies in regards to the health and longevity of cellular life. They've confirmed that if both the outside and inside environment of a cell is kept clean and undefiled, as long as the cell is washed continuously with pure distilled water, nourished properly, and the condition both inside and outside the cell remains uncontaminated, that cell can live forever without breaking down or aging. The cell will continue to regenerate itself without losing elasticity or developing disease. I have had so many people casually say to me, it doesn't matter what I eat. They have this huge disconnection between the food they eat and what it can do to their bodies. Look at what weird things can happen when we allow our inside environments to become defiled. Recently, scientists made a surprising discovery that even baffled the veterans. After more than 20 years of examining salmon, something mysteriously strange started happening. All of the male salmon had freakishly developed female and male reproductive organs, while all the female salmon's reproductive organs remained unchanged.

The scientists could not believe what they were finding and immediately started an intensive investigation. What they learned was that the water these fish lived in had unusually high levels of estrogen, a mostly female hormone. Scientists noted that the recent use of estrogen by women to treat hormonal imbalances had greatly increased over the years. Mysteriously, water from industrialized cities had reached the local tributaries which contaminated the fish's ecosystem. These fish then ate the food contaminated with estrogen and this eventually brought about metabolic changes, causing them to develop female reproductive organs. This incident undeniably verifies the fact that what goes into your body can cause major changes, good or bad. Our fruits and vegetables contain both vitamins, minerals, antioxidants, and pure water distilled naturally by nature through the soil. Our cells are nourished by these same life-sustaining nutrients, while at the same time, the distilled water oxygenates, washes, and cleanses our cellular environments.

What an awesome and mighty God we serve. How could anyone have ever imagined something as complex as this to have evolved through the process of evolution? How could the fruit ever have known that its primary mission would involve washing and nourishing the cellular ecosystem of mankind, to promote health, healing, and longevity? Fruit is not intelligent nor does it have the ability to think on its' own, or does it? After all, it was ordained by God to fulfill its purpose, and just maybe it listens and obeys God more than we do. It appears as if the trees and fruits in nature are actually healthier than we are. What's also interesting to note is the fact that our bodies and fruit have a very similar composition, mostly water and minerals from which we were both created. Both man and fruit decompose and return back to dust of the earth after death in pretty much the same manner.

The water in our fruits and vegetables is naturally distilled by the soil as long as the soil remains undefiled. Does not this picture of cellular health and disease-free longevity mentioned earlier remind us of the new heaven and earth described in the book of Revelation, Chapter 22? There it describes a pure river of water, clear as crystal, proceeding out of the throne of God and the Lamb. It further states in chapter 21:27, that nothing that defileth shall be allowed to enter into this new kingdom. There will be nothing allowed in that can cause sickness, disease, or death.

The Tree of Life mentioned in Chapter 22 will be nourished with pure, crystal clear water. Both the air and soil will be pure, because they will both consist of and exist of God Himself. Every person allowed in will be pure with pure motives, pure ideas, pure thoughts, pure conversation, pure songs, and a pure new glorified body. I get excited just thinking about the fact that we will finally be able to live in perpetual peace and happiness. No more foul language, foul music, foul attitudes, or foul people. The fruit from the Tree of Life will be totally pure and undefiled by toxic chemicals and fertilizers. No one will selfishly try to turn a profit by harvesting the fruit before it has ripened. Revelation 2:7 says, "He who has an ear, let him hear what the spirit says to the churches. To him who overcomes I will give to eat from the Tree of Life, which is in the midst of the Paradise of God." This is the same tree that Adam and Eve were prevented from eating before being evicted from the Garden of Eden.

The fruit from the Tree of the Knowledge of Good and Evil was never meant to be eaten, but here we see under the right conditions, the Tree of Life was allowed to be eaten. In other words, had Adam and Eve overcame their temptation in the Garden of Eden, and remained unscarred by sin, they would have been allowed to eat from the Tree of Life and experience eternal life and physical well being. This trait then possessed by Adam and Eve would have been passed down to all of their offspring, even right down to us today. Of course, God had no intention of sin existing forever, which would have been the case had they eaten from the Tree of Life in their sinful state. Notice what Genesis 3:22-24 says, "Then the Lord God said, behold the man has become like one of us, to know good and evil. And now, lest he put out his hand and take from the Tree of Life, and eat, and live forever. 23. therefore the lord God sent him out of the Garden of Eden to till the ground from which he was taken. 24. So he drove out the man; and he placed cherubim at the east of the Garden of Eden, and a flaming sword which turned every way, to guard the way to the Tree of Life."

This is the same Tree of Life now mentioned in the book of Revelation, but no longer protected by the cherubim who guarded it against Adam and Eve. Those who do not overcome will be cast into the Lake of Fire and not allowed to eat from the Tree of Life, so they will suffer sickness and disease throughout their eternal existence. However, believers will enjoy perfect health and eternal longevity sustained by the leaves from the Tree of Life. Revelation 22:2 states that "the leaves of the tree were for the healing of the nations." God has placed seed bearing herbs on the earth to heal diseases, and seed bearing fruits to promote health and wellness. The fruit and leaves from the Tree of Life will promote both health and longevity. I don't want to crash anyone's party here, but it appears as though God has already determined the menu that will be served in heaven. So if you're planning on a seafood festival, a pig roast, or eating hamburgers and fries, you're in for a big surprise. Relax! You can laugh, it's okay!!!! You are fearfully and wonderfully created to fulfill God's plans in the earth and for no other reason.

Don't get it wrong- you were not created to serve your own purpose or interest, but to serve God's purpose only. Your body, He wonderfully and masterfully crafted with remarkable durability, is proof of this concept. Look how God created you with trillions of self regenerating and self-repairing cells, tissue, and organs. He made sure you were equipped with more than enough cells to compensate for the mistakes and abuse we would subject ourselves to throughout our lives. God knew that we would accidentally and ignorantly destroy almost half of our cells through a lifestyle of partying, drinking, substance abuse, and unhealthy eating habits. God foreknew that Satan would infiltrate our food supply, and for the love of money, poison it. He knew that we would be misguided and misinformed about nutrition as it relates to the temple where the Holy Spirit dwells.

He supplied us with more than enough cells than we would ever need. In fact, humans only use 10% to 20% percent of their brain's total capacity their entire lifetime. Moreover, just in case our internal systems became inoperable due to cell degeneration, He placed healing powers in herbs, fruits, and vegetables to repair and promote wellness in our bodies. During the bubonic plague that hit Europe, four thieves were caught stealing from the homes of those who had succumb to the deadly virus. Although the virus was highly contagious, these thieves never became sick, even though they were eating and drinking the food from the homes of the deceased. After being caught and interrogated by authorities, the thieves revealed that they had eaten and rubbed raw garlic all over their bodies and clothing. Today, scientists have confirmed that garlic is one of the greatest potent natural antibiotics. Garlic promotes cell health and works to help clean up our cellular environments. More is explained about the remarkable benefits of garlic in **Chapter 12.**

Now it's up to us to make sure that our internal cellular environments are kept viable and healthy. Paul teaches us in 1st Corinthians that our bodies belong to God, that we were bought and purchased at a price. This body or temple that houses our soul and spirit is simply on loan to us, as we travel on a round trip assignment from heaven, through earth and then back to heaven. In other words, while we physically exist in this present age, everything in the universe is on loan to us: the sun, moon, clouds, water, wind, rain, etc. When we complete our assignment and depart this temporary present age, we take nothing with us, not even the dust of the ground from which we come. A good example of this is like taking a round trip flight on an airplane. While in the air, everything inside the universe of the plane is on loan to you like the seats, pillows, floatation devices, and even the pilot and crew. However, once your trip is over, you take none of these things with you as you depart the plane.

While living in this present age, since spirits are invisible in this worldly material realm, they must occupy earthly material to become physically visible. Jesus had to take on earthly material in the form of a physical body, in order to live and dwell amongst mankind. The material body He occupied while living on this earth was on loan to Him. While occupying this body, tent, or temple, He fulfilled the plans of His father here on the earth. Jesus willingly submitted His will to that of the Father, and totally honored God with all of His body, mind, soul, and spirit. If we are to truly live by the examples that Christ has set before us, we must do the same. The scientific and medical community are in total agreement with the Bible in regards to health and nutrition. Medical science has concluded that 75% of all degenerative diseases are directly caused by unhealthy eating habits, lack of exercise, and smoking. These are all habits of choice, and unfortunately, they are the main culprit causing the majority of our illnesses.

Now let's go to the Bible for confirmation. Deuteronomy 30:19 says, "I have set before you life and death, blessing and cursing: therefore choose life, that both thou and thy seed may live." Here again we are still dealing with choices, both the Bible and science seem to conclude that if the right choices are made, one can definitely live and not just live, but live with health and vitality. Both the Bible and science are saying you don't have to suffer with degenerative diseases. All of the money believers are allowing the enemy to take from the kingdom of God through our health can be reversed. The unnecessary suffering we are experiencing can be alleviated and undone. The choices and the decisions are set before you. No on is going to force you. You have to take the right action for yourself. Make a conscious decision and ask yourself, do you love satisfying and honoring the desires of your flesh more than you love honoring God?

There are three Hebrew words I want to explain to you as they relate to the creation of mankind. These words will confirm and attest to the Apostle Paul's statement in regards to our bodies belonging to God, and not ourselves. In <u>Genesis 1:27 it says, "So God created (bara) man in His own image, in the image of God he created he him, male and female created he them.</u>" The Hebrew word for created here is (bara) to bring into being. Here a new form of spiritual life (soul and spirit) to be occupied in an earthly material body is brought into existence represented by mankind. Up until this point, God hadn't created a soul and spirit to occupy a fleshly earthly body. Next <u>Genesis 2:7 it says, "And the Lord God formed (yatsar) man of the dust of the ground, and breathed into his nostrils the breath of life, and man became a living soul."</u> The Hebrew word here for <u>formed</u> is (<u>yatsar</u>), to mold or squeeze into shape as a potter does with clay when he is shaping and forming pottery. So in Chapter One, the immaterial invi-sible soul and spirit (the inner man) were created (<u>bara</u>) first, and then in Chapter Two, the visible physical body, tent, temple, or hous-ing was formed (<u>yatsar</u>) from a mixture of dust (dry land /new begin-ning) and water. This earthly temple, tent, or house would serve as temporary residence for the new spirit man, enabling him to occupy physical space in the earthly realm.

<u>Psalms 24:1 says "The earth is the Lord's and all its fullness the world and those who dwell therein."</u> God took what was His by divine authority, and created our bodies out of what belonged and yet belongs to Himself, and never once did He state that we belong to ourselves. Notice how the spiritual man was created and the physical body was formed, both existing separately, yet neither possessed life in and of themselves. God decided to fearfully and wonderfully fuse the two together, breathe into this union the breath of life, and they became one living being. God united the spirit with the body, performed the very first marriage ceremony, and then blessed this union.

Let's take a moment here and examine the complexity and awesomeness of our earthly temple. We were truly fearfully and won-derfully created for a purpose, and not just by accident or by chance. Our heart beats 4,200 times an hour, and pumps 12 tons of blood daily. In a 24-hour period, the 600,000,000 air cells located in our lungs inhale 2,400 gallons of air. There are roughly 20,000 hairs located in the ear to tune in sound, and over 20,000,000 mouths that suck food as it travels through our intestines. We have a delicate web of 10 million or so nerves and extensions, intertwined through 600 muscles wrapped around 263 bones, and we can't leave out the 970 miles of blood vessels. Our internal communications system runs circles around all of the combined cell phone and satellite companies on the planet by allowing us to talk to persons they'll never be able to reach- our heavenly Father, His son Christ Jesus, and the precious Holy Spirit.

This detailed description of God's intricate involvement in the creation and fusing together of the spirit and body totally disproves the theory of evolution. No evolutionary process could have accidentally created and formed mankind, joined together the spirit, soul, and body, given them life, and then ultimately bless this new creation. Furthermore, Genesis 2:22 says, "And the rib, which the Lord had taken from man, made (panah) he woman, and brought her unto the man." The Hebrew word made here is (panah) to be skillfully formed or fashioned, and not (bara) the word God used to form the body of man. In other words, God took His time while creating the body, tent, or temple to house the woman that he took out of the man. He paid very close attention to detail, and rather skillfully built her a body, while the body made for the man was simply squeezed into shape. This could explain why men and women are so different in character. Men will come home from work dirty and soiled without really being too bothered or concerned. Just give him his favorite chair, remote control, and a TV dinner, and he's good to go. Women, on the other hand, are normally neater and cleaner than men. They like to shower up and refresh themselves, before getting up-close and personal. They don't like the thought of keeping on dirty clothes and especially not laying around in them which for a man, is not such a big deal. Of course there are some exceptions to this rule, and the opposite can be true for both sexes in some cases.

As I stated earlier, there is nothing we can really do concerning the nature of our outside environments. However, you can make informed and educated decisions about what you allow to enter your inner cellular environment. For example, the cancer epidemic being played out in our society is not being caused by people who are intentionally exposing themselves to radioactive material. Who in their right mind would do such a foolish thing? As a matter of fact, the average sane person does all that is within their power to avoid nuclear waste. Crowds of people are not traveling out of their way to nuclear power plants, seeking to purchase uranium for personal consumption or to feed to their children. Even in hospitals, extra care is taken to cover patients with protective garments to reduce or eliminate the exposure to radiation emitted by the x-ray machines. The person administering the test is usually hiding behind a protective barrier of some sort. Most of the radioactive material in this country is heavily guarded 24 hours a day by sophisticated computers, elaborate security measures, heavily armed guards, and highly trained protection dogs.

So as you can plainly see, we are not getting cancer from our outside environment. It is too heavily protected. The only other way we can develop cancer in such epidemic proportions is if our inside environment is continuously contaminated by what we expose it to. Now that's exactly what's happening. We're defiling ourselves through our unhealthy eating habits and sedentary lifestyles. We are exposing our internal environment to things and conditions that promote the development of degenerative diseases and sicknesses such as cancer. In fact, this is even further confirmed by the fact that most cancers are reversible if caught in their earliest stages. This is why proper cell health is so important, because they have the remarkable ability to regenerate after their own kind.

Almost ten years ago, I met a young lady who was literally on her death bed. She had been suffering for many years without any clue as to what was causing her acute illness. Even after being examined by doctors from coast to coast, her mysterious illness could not be properly diagnosed. None of the medications worked in reversing or curing her excruciatingly painful condition. So she was sent home without any hope, to simply waste away and die. Her husband stood by and helplessly watched as she suffered and her health slowly deteriorated. With a death sentence from the doctors, and no relief from her medications, she decided to turn to the Lord. This turning point literally saved her life, because it put her on a quest to seek alternative methods of treatment. What she learned would shock everyone, including her doctors. She changed her eating habits and for six months, all she ate was broccoli, baked potatoes, drank plenty of water, natural juicing, and took herbs. In just a couple months, her illness had totally cleared up and she was no longer on her death bed. The painful condition that had plagued her body for years was suddenly gone, and all she had to do was make some healthier lifestyle choices. Today, she is full of health and vitality, and to look at her, you would never know that she had ever been so close to death.

In the end, it was determined that she had not been drinking enough water, and had developed hundreds of gallstones. This one condition debilitated her entire body and forced it to begin shutting down. Listen, drinking coffee and soda will not take the place of clean water, because both of these drinks actually dehydrate the body and leach minerals from the bones. Clean, distilled water is best for humans and is absolutely needed to properly hydrate the bodies cellular environments. In fact, she told me that she never drank water because she didn't feel it was that important. So for years, her cells were unable to receive proper cleansing and flushing. They were unable to receive fresh oxygen, nutrients, minerals, and transfer vital information. She dehydrated herself and deprived her cells of valuable oxygen. This extended putrefying environment ultimately brought about her unnecessary suffering and almost premature death.

So many people casually say to me all the time that they do not drink water, and it totally amazes me. Imagine never taking a bath in fresh clean water, but the same old dirty bath water every day for several years. Now envision over 80 trillion cells swimming in this dirty, filthy, highly acidic, and toxic environment. These are your cells which make up every part of your body. This would almost be equivalent to a person using the same toilet, day in and day out, for several years but never flushing it. Now here's the real kicker. You get to leave the restroom after you use it, but your cells never get to travel outside of their horrific deteriorating environment. They are eternally locked in with no way of escape. These cells start regenerating unhealthy mutagent cells which attack the weakest organs in the body. For her, it was the gall bladder. She had developed hundreds of gallstones that were being misdiagnosed, causing doctors to prescribe the wrong medications which weren't working, when all she really needed was pure water and internal cleansing and hydration.

The human body is comprised of 75% water, is amazingly resilient, and has the inherent power and ability to regenerate and repair itself whenever necessary. In order to accomplish these monumental tasks, it must always stay properly hydrated with water, not soda or coffee. As I speak, a majority of the people living in this country are mineral-depleted and totally dehydrated. The human skeleton consists of 35% water and 40% mineral composition. Without this complex combination kept in constant balance, our bones become weak and brittle causing us to develop all kinds of bone degenerating diseases such as osteoporosis.

Often times when people hear the word tumor, they cringe and the big letter "C" immediately pops into their minds. Fortunately, every tumor is not malignant or cancerous, and if dealt with in a timely fashion, are completely harmless. In fact, the formation of a tumor is good and can be lifesaving. Tumors are actually the body's defense mechanism that helps protect your vital organs, allowing them to continue functioning while you get needed help. To a certain degree, tumors and fat can be your friend and your enemy all at the same time. For example, a tumor is really just dangerous waste materials in the body that have been localized, entombed, and pushed aside. Basically, they collect dangerous waste materials, entomb them, and tuck them somewhere out of the way. This prevents it from spreading throughout the body, allowing you to continue functioning, giving you the time you need to correct the situation. What a mighty God we serve!

In a way, a tumor is a good sign, because it means that there is a system failure taking place within the body, and for the time being, the body is dealing with it. Fat surrounding the vital organs sort of acts the same way in that it also serves as protection when the body remains in an extended period of toxicity. Your major internal organs, like the liver, kidneys, heart, etc., are vitally important to your survival. When the body is in a toxic condition, these internal organs will produce and enclose themselves in extra fat. This procedure allows the bacteria, molds, fungi, and parasites to feed on the fat while the vital organ stays safe and able to function, providing protection for the organs. If they didn't surround and enclose themselves within fat, an army of deadly invaders would attack, thus totally disabling them and causing premature death. If this situation is not reversed through proper cleansing, followed by healthy lifestyle choices, it can start the onset of degenerative diseases.

There is a disease called NASH, which stands for Non-Alcoholic Steatorrhoeic Hepatosis, that severely affects the health and function of the liver. Since the liver plays such a major role in the overall function of the body, this condition, if not treated, can contribute to a whole host of degenerative diseases to include liver failure and, ultimately, death.

This disease is when the liver becomes overwhelmed with fat and actually turns into a big sack of fat. In this condition, the liver can not make bile to clean the blood nor can it burn fat. So someone suffering with this ailment can experience difficulty controlling their weight, always feeling tired, elevated cholesterol levels, and even diabetes. Look at how just one impaired organ can cause system failures in other organs. Every cell is linked together and so is every organ. You can't take out your heart, and expect the rest of the body to keep on functioning. You must keep the entire body cleansed and undefiled to the best of your ability. Now when it does happen to get contaminated, eating and drinking alkalizing foods and herbs is the only way to get the body back to optimum health. Conventional medicine is not the answer to metabolic degenerative diseases like diabetes, hypertension, cancer, obesity, and heart disease. Lifestyle changes and constant internal cleansing and detoxing will have lasting, positive affects.

I once helped a 58-year-old gentleman who was suffering with high cholesterol, diabetes, obesity, and was using two inhalers. He had been using Lipitor to treat his high cholesterol. Soon after we met, he was also diagnosed with prostate cancer. He immediately made lifestyle changes and upon later diagnosis, all of these conditions had completely cleared up. In fact, he no longer needed the use of his inhalers which he had used for several years. I know you think this is exciting but it gets even better. This man had used illicit drugs for almost thirty years of his life combined with unhealthy eating habits. This story serves as a real testament to the validity of the word of God. After thirty years of abuse and neglect, you would expect for his body to be unresponsive and impaired. In less than six months, not only had his body responded, but it also totally healed itself. Currently, he's working on losing an additional ten pounds and admits, he has never felt better in his life. Once while coming down with the symptoms of a cold, he used an all-natural approach, and within two days, the symptoms were gone. What really shocked him was the fact that the cold never fully developed; he just experienced the symptoms.

The word of God doesn't need to be proven or researched. God has ordained all of creation by his word, and this is why after thirty years of neglect and abuse, his body still responded as soon as he changed his lifestyle. Conventional medicines could have never produced these results, because they are acidic and only mask the symptoms. In fact, up until the time we met, he had no idea that an all-natural solution could help his condition. Medications are created by man and all come with warnings of potentially fatal side affects, which disproves its effectiveness. The workout guru Jack Lalane once stated, if man made it don't eat it. He's almost 100 years old and still works out regularly.

The law does not allow us to use counterfeit money. Why should we settle for a counterfeit healing? Only what God has ordained can He backup and maintain, to effectively and thoroughly bring about total deliverance and recovery. You are fearfully and wonderfully made, and this is why his body responded so well after 30 years. If this man can make lifestyle changes and it worked for him, you should take notice and decide to save your health and your loved ones. **Remember, God has placed before you life and death, sickness and disease, so choose life, that you and your seed may live.**

C H A P T E R   5

The Real Time Bomb
"Hydrogenated Oils"

"I have set before you life and death, blessing and cursing: therefore choose life, that both thou and thy seed may live:" (Deuteronomy 30:19)

Nearly 75 years ago while experimenting in a laboratory, a group of scientists put on their thinking caps and came to the conclusion that mankind's almost 4,400-year-old diet, which God had commanded to Noah following the great flood, was no longer safe for his health. Genesis 9:1-3, "So God blessed Noah and his sons, and said to them, be fruitful and multiply, and fill the earth. (2) And the fear of you and the dread of you shall be on every beast of the earth, on every bird of the air, on all that move on the earth, and on all flesh of the sea, they are given onto your hand. (3) Every moving thing that lives shall be food for you. I have given you all things, even as the green herbs." Here, for the first time, the mention of moving creatures being considered as food for mankind is introduced, as well as the first declaration of all things given to mankind for food, making reference to the green herbs, the second dietary command communicated by God in Genesis 3:18. Verse 3 indicates mankind's third and final dietary instructions that have lasted since the time of Noah. Also revealed here is the initial fear and dread that all creatures would now have of mankind, explaining how Noah was able to peacefully live with the animals aboard the ark, and the animals even coming aboard in the first place.

Unlike cattle ranchers of today, Noah didn't have to rope all the animals like a herdsmen. They entered the ark on their own without being afraid. Imagine Noah chasing after rabbits, gazelles, and cheetahs who can run up to 75 miles per hour. Picture him trying to catch these wild animals at 600 years of age. I'm already out of breath at just the thought, and I'm only 40; that's 560 years younger than he was. Okay, stop laughing. I was only kidding, and you thought it was funny. Anyway, these scientists determined that since this 4,400 year old diet consisted of saturated fats derived from the consumption of animal flesh, it had to be unhealthy for the human heart and arteries, because it raised the levels of fat and cholesterol present in the blood. Remember <u>Leviticus 17:11 says, "the Life of the flesh is in the blood."</u> So these highly educated and astute scientists decided that we needed a healthier source of fats in our diets, one that would be heart healthier and friendly. In other words, they were trying to reverse what God had intentionally allowed to evolve. You see, God shortened man's life intentionally for mankind's own safety and for the preservation of the earth. <u>Genesis 6:5 says, "and God saw that the wickedness of man was great in the earth, and that every imagination of the thoughts of his heart was only evil continually."</u> Verse 6 states, that it grieved God's heart that he had made man. Although mankind didn't eat from the Tree of Life mentioned in Genesis 2:9, and receive the reward of eternal physical longevity, he was actually able to live a long and healthy life in his violent transgressions.

Verse 7 further states that since the iniquities of mankind had reached heaven, God made the decision to wipe every living creature off the face of the earth. So between the fall of mankind and the great flood, had mankind been able to live without so much evil in his heart, God would have never needed to shorten his life. By allowing mankind to eat meat, his life would shorten; thus, he would live a curtailed, less destructive time on the earth. We know today that meat consumption is linked to heart disease, cancer, hypertension, kidney failure, obesity, gout, arthritis, and a plethora of chronic afflictions. Meat also robs the body of energy during digestion, elevates levels of excess cholesterol, plaque, and fat present in the blood, which is life in the flesh.

All of these factors greatly contribute to the shortening of one's life and greatly contributes to cell degradation. Instead of extinguishing mankind, God found favor in Noah and destroyed all but Noah and his family, which brings us to why God introduced meat into the new covenant He established with Noah following the flood. Since God had blessed the image He created of Himself, He couldn't go back on His words and utterly wipe us out. So the same animals whose blood had been used to atone for the sins of mankind in Genesis 4:4 would now be used to shorten his life of evil and corruption. This is exactly what happened immediately following this epochal event.

So armed with credentials and the profundity of their intellience, these brilliant minds took it upon themselves to create a healthier fat than what God had given to mankind since the great flood. Remember, originally animal flesh was not a part of man's initial diet, according to Genesis 1:29; 3:18; 4:4:and 9:3. Up until this point, he had only eaten herbs, fruits, seeds, nuts, and vegetables. The seeds and vegetables contained essential fatty acids most suited for human beings, preventing cancer and heart disease. The absence of animal flesh explains one of the reasons why the patriarchs lived for so long and in such good health. Immediately following the introduction of animal flesh into mankind's diet, the life span of humans fell precipitously by more than 700 years in just nine generations. Genesis 11:32 says, "So the days of Terah were two hundred and five years, and Terah died in Haran." So Terah, being nine generations from Adam, was the last of the patriarchs to live past the age of 200.

I know many of you are probably asking about Job who was given an extra 140 years to live. Many scholars agree that Job more than likely lived in the patriarchal days due to the fact that he acted in the role of a priest by offering up sacrifices acceptable to God to atone for the sins of his family. Job 1:5 says, "So it was when the days of festival had run their course, that Job would send and sanctify them, and he would rise early in the morning and offer burnt offerings according to the number of them all. For Job said, it may be that my sons have sinned and cursed God in their hearts. This Job did regularly." This practice was common during the days of the patriarchs, before God initiated the priestly order through Aaron, Moses' brother. Remember the books of the Bible are not placed in chronological order. You can read the Reese Chronological Bible for a better understanding of times, dates, and events in the Bible.

So without consulting God or getting His permission, these scientists set out to experiment in a laboratory and create an all-new synthetically man-made fat called "trans fats." From the manipulation of hydrogen gas and fats contained in vegetable oils, trans fats are made when hydrogenated gas is fused into the oils using a metal catalyst, aluminum, cobalt, and nickel, converting the oils from a liquid into a solid. Without the metals, the hydrogen could not be fused into the oils. All of these metals are toxic, throwing the body's pH out of balance. This fusion takes place under pressure at temperatures of 250-400 degrees Celsius. When you compare these transformed essential fatty acids which have now become a trans-fatty acid, it is analogous with the molecular structure of stearic acid. Stearic acid has many uses, one of which is in the making of candles. It causes the candles to harden. This action is probably replicated in the arteries of humans causing them to harden, leading to heart disease or arteriosclerosis. A Harvard Medical School study followed more than 85,000 women over an eight-year period. The researchers compared the diets of those who developed heart disease over that time with those who did not. They found that major dietary sources of trans-fats, such as margarine, were significantly associated with higher risks of coronary heart disease.

Deaths from heart disease have now surpassed over 750,000 lives a year. Before the introduction of this counterfeit fat into our food supply, heart disease as we know it, was rare in this country. The fusing of particular metals such as aluminum into the oils could well be the reason today why people are being detected with high levels of aluminum. It is thought that aluminum has been implicated in causing Alzheimer's disease, cancer, complications associated with both Type I and Type II diabetes and lead poisoning in children. Non-radioactive cobalt, the kind used as a catalyst in these oils, is a component of Vitamin B12. Many studies have suggested that large amounts of this type of cobalt can cause cell disintegration and nerve disorders. Further, the fatty acids have been transformed molecularly so that the body doesn't know how to correctly metabolize them. In other words, the scientists were trying to perform a marriage of molecules that only God had the authority to do and could ordain to properly function inside the human body.

Hydrogenated oils have the remarkable ability to prevent spoilage, keeping foods fresh in the packages for many years, and in some cases, even decades. It also has the added benefit of making baked and fried foods look and taste better by making them crispier and crunchier. Does this not remind us of <u>Genesis 3:6 "So when the woman saw that the tree was good for food, that it was pleasant to</u>

the eyes, and a tree desirable to make one wise, she took of its fruit and ate." This new fat was widely introduced to the general public as margarine in 1936. Crisco oil, Mazola oils, and a host of other refined and hydrogenated products began to make significant penetration into the food markets of the nation. Support for dairy and opposition to margarine faded during World War II due to butter shortages. So the dairy industry began focusing primarily on supplying the military, while the rest of the general public was furnished margarine, and products containing hydrogenated oils from food processing companies.

It was touted by the medical and scientific community as being a new heart-healthy fat that could even protect against heart disease. Before long, margarine was out selling real butter, which had been around for hundreds of years. What's also interesting to note is that 75 years ago, the major cause of death was not heart disease, but infectious diseases like malaria, small pox, measles, chicken pox, and polio. At the turn of the century, deaths resulting from heart disease, stroke, cancer, and diabetes were very rare. In fact, these diseases were virtually unheard of, and Type II diabetes didn't even exist. Around this same time, the incidence of diabetes and its associated diseases were diagnosed at around 2.8% per 100,000 of the population. Over the last fifty years and since the introduction of hydrogenated oils, this disease has increased over 2000%.

There were also two other epochal events during this same period that, in my opinion, contributed to the sudden hike in degenerative related diseases. They include the increased consumption of refined sugar in this country and the widespread use of mineral depleted salt. This salt, called table salt, contains highly poisonous aluminum and other by-products that inhibit proper digestion. None of these three substances occur naturally anywhere in nature and are a deadly concoction. Three dangerous counterfeits of guerrilla warfare introduced into our food supply around the same time. I think the adversary drew up this battle plan to cripple and utterly destroy the image that God placed of Himself into this present age of the betrayer. Soon after food production companies started using hydrogenated oils, substantial increases in several diseases occurred within a few years.

During the late1930's and early1940's, a dramatic increase was seen in the following diseases. First was a disease that looked like diabetes, but was not caused by a deficiency of insulin. The medical profession was dumbfounded. All they knew was that a person produced enough insulin, but it was not effective in reducing sugar in the blood. They did not know what caused the insulin to be resistant. The medical establishment named this new disease non-insulin dependent diabetes, Type II. The second and third diseases that increased dramatically were heart disease and cancer. Today, cancer is the number one killer of all people under the age of 85 in this country. Those under 85 comprise 98.4% percent of the total population. That means that only the very oldest Americans (2.6%) continue to die of heart disease more so than of cancer, a trend that is expected to reverse by 2018. A third of all cancers are related to smoking, and another two thirds are related to obesity, poor diet and lack of exercise, all factors that also contribute to heart disease. Deaths from colon cancer and lung cancer in men are particularly striking. They're dropping so fast that they exceed the impact of aging, which increases the likelihood of developing cancer, according to Dr. Harmon Eyre, the American Cancer Society's long-time chief medical officer.

This is also the period where new diseases, which fell into the autoimmune classifications, were being seen for the first time and named. The medical profession also did not know what was causing these new autoimmune diseases. They placed blame on the faulty genetics of the immune system. The connection here is that the increase of these new diseases began shortly after the introduction of hydrogenated oils in the food supply. Here we have another counterfeit substance, just like sugar, both being synthetic and both appealing to taste. Both causing catastrophic disease and premature death as if someone had actually dropped a real hydrogen bomb into our bodies. It again appears as though we should have taken our cue from the animals. For you see, no animal, insect, not even bacteria will eat margarine, which is why it has such a long shelf life.

There was a story about some Hostess Twinkies that had been floating around for almost 30 years, and were still fresh in the package. I have had cookies, crackers, cakes, etc. hang out in the cupboards for years and never rot. This isn't normal with natural foods, because if you notice they start to spoil within just a few days. However back to the animals, insects, and bacteria. Why won't they touch this stuff? I mean it seems as though flies will eat just about anything, even a decomposing horse and its feces. Molds and bacteria anxiously wait in line for their shot to takeover. Yet none of these creatures will eat margarine or go near it. Hog farmers won't even feed trans-fatty acid foods or hydrogenated oiled foods to their hogs. The reason is because hogs will die when eating these oils, and hogs will eat anything, including dead rats.

However, highly intelligent humans consume this garbage by the tons every year. Since the introduction of this hydrogen bomb into our food supply, the rate of degenerative diseases has risen in direct proportion to its increased consumption. Today, heart disease is the number one killer of woman, and is the leading cause of all deaths in North America, Canada, and Europe. Dr. Lenore Kohlmeier in Finland completed a study on 700 women, 300 of them had breast cancer. The study included analysis of cells from the fat tissue of these women. Dr. Kohlmeier issued this statement, "women who have higher stores of trans-fatty acids have a 1.4 times (nearly a 55%) higher risk of developing breast cancer." Harvard researchers published their findings stating that, "it's not the level of or amount of fat intake that increases heart attacks and heart disease, but the type of fats consumed, especially trans-fatty acids." Studies show conclusively that trans-fatty oils cause Type II diabetes, and this disease can eventually burn out the pancreas resulting in Type I diabetes.

These counterfeit oils dramatically increase the risk of arteriosclerosis, breast cancer, various types of cancers and autoimmune diseases. Over 100 research studies reveal the extent to which these oils greatly harm the human body. One hundred years ago, heart disease was all but unknown. Today, two-thirds of US citizens develop heart disease. So it appears as if this new healthier fat touted as being heart healthy was actually heart deadly. 1st Corinthians 1:19 says, "For it is written, I will destroy the wisdom of the wise, and will bring to nothing the understanding of the prudent." By the way, as I am writing this book, a very small amount of trans fats are quietly being removed from our food supply. You may have even noticed lately new labeling on some of the grocery items you normally purchase. They either say "no trans fats" or "non hydrogenated oils."

Why is there all of a sudden an urgent need to remove this hydrogen bomb from our food supply? Because the FDA has already warned that this counterfeit fat is dangerous for human consumption. By 2006, the USDA has mandated that this toxic poisonous bomb be listed on all food labels. Since it is no longer good for your health, a warning label will more than likely be required. So the food industry is trying to stay one step ahead by quietly removing some of this deadly hydrogen bomb from the food supply. Listen, don't get too relaxed, not even for one second, because with all of the other junk in our food supply, you are far from being safe and out of the woods. The potential loss of billions of dollars by food processors and patent owners if this deadly oil was removed from what we consume has kept it in our food supply to date. Essential fatty acids are the building blocks of fats.

They play important roles within the human body by affecting almost every major organ, like cell membrane production and immune system function. Natural occurring essential fatty acids have an electrical weight that charges the fluidity of cell membranes. This is very important on how healthy immune cells develop. When oils are transformed by the hydrogenation process, this electrical weight is changed in essential fatty acids. This affects the fluidity which causes cell membranes to stiffen.

Here's one little secret the food industry forgot to let us in on... that they had plans to put this garbage into everything we eat. That's right, up to 95% of all processed foods and restaurant foods contain trans fatty oils in them. In all actuality, foods containing hydrogenated oils should be removed from every grocery shelf in America. The next time you go shopping, just read the ingredients listed on the foods you buy and you will find it everywhere.

Why am I making such a big fuss about hydrogenated oils? Remember I mentioned before that your body's pH level must remain balanced in order to maintain optimum cellular health. What takes your body out of balance is the level of potential hydrogen atoms present in the blood at any given time. If you have high levels of hydrogen atoms in the blood, the amount of available oxygen is greatly reduced. Leviticus 17:11 says, "For the Life of the flesh is in the blood." Your cells breathe in oxygen in the same way your lungs breath in oxygen. With the reduction in available oxygen, your cells are unable to communicate with each other because they are starving for oxygen. Imagine for a moment only knowing how to speak English then suddenly being placed in China. You would find it very difficult, if not impossible, trying to live and communicate with the local population who now overcrowd your environment. The language barrier would be a major handicap hampering your ability to get things done like banking, shopping, and other normal daily tasks. At this point, you would have three options, either leave the country, learn the language, or hire an interpreter.

I once walked into a grocery store in Southern California because I was hungry and wanted to buy something to eat. I couldn't buy anything in the store because all the ingredients on the labels were listed in Chinese. Trying to understand Chinese was totally alien to me because I had never spoken or learned the language in my entire life. I could not believe how difficult it was for me to find something in the store I could understand. Because I'm always checking food labels, I wasn't about to eat anything I couldn't read. I was finally forced to leave and go to a store where I could understand the ingredients listed on the label. The reality of this major communication barrier really hit hard, and it still bothers me to this day.

Now let's return back to the human body and see how communication barriers can cause havoc and major dysfunctions. Without being able to communicate, the cells can't carry the proper information to other cells, that speak to other organs that activate different types of bodily functions, like the release of hormones into the blood. The cells become confused and disorientated in the same way flight crews and passengers can lose consciousness if there is a sudden drop in air cabin pressure during a flight. The aircraft is pressurized to maintain the right level of oxygen at high altitudes where there is not enough breathable oxygen. Pilots can become confused, disorientated, and can fall unconscious in as little as two minutes if cabin pressure suddenly drops. Without immediate action taken to get fresh oxygen, the pilot will lose consciousness and the plane will crash, not reaching its intended destination. The air traffic controllers will not be able to help the pilot, because the lack of oxygen has made effective communication next to impossible. This once safe and normal flight has now become dangerous and deadly, because the pilot has become incapacitated due to lack of oxygen. Everyone on the plane must suffer the consequences that could result in the plane crashing, taking the lives of all onboard.

When your cells can't communicate with your organs, your whole body must pay the cost. Your body starts to develop symptoms of this condition which leads to metabolic degenerative disorders like diabetes, heart disease, cancer, obesity, high blood pressure, and a host of other complications. This oxygen-deprived environment causes our cells to become confused. Your cells are normally oval shaped and very pliable. They fit into each other a certain way in order to communicate the needed information for vital bodily functions. Trans-fatty oils stiffen the outer cellular membrane and weakens the structural integrity of the cell. This alters normal transport of minerals and other nutrients across the cell membrane, and allows disease microbes and toxic chemicals to get into the cell more easily. The end result is trillions of diseased, ineffective cells, faulty organ capacity and immune system dysfunction. This compromised state of affairs decreases immunity and increases susceptibility to illness.

The fact that only humans will eat this garbage proves that the independent internal instinct given to the animals by God still works very well today. Some people don't have a bowel movement for 3 to 4 days at a time because their cells can't communicate the need to pass out waste. When the cells become deformed in shape, communication is all but impossible. Without communication, proper cell division and regeneration is also impossible. Cells begin to pass along the wrong information. Once this happens, you now have new degenerating cells that haven't received the right information, so they start mutating into alien cells.

This is why cancer cells are so hard to destroy and can live forever, because they didn't receive the right information from the cell before it. They don't know that they're supposed to get along peaceably with other cells, and eventually die according to their life's clock cycle. This life clock cycle contains the expiration date of every healthy cell. Since this pertinent information is never passed on to cancerous cells, they can't pass it on to other cells. Instead of dying, they just keep on living and multiplying, attacking as well as destroying normal healthy cells in the body. While your normal cells are dying based on their life's clock cycle, and being prematurely destroyed by the mutating alien cancerous cells, these cancerous cells continue mutating into other types of cells and multiplying, until you have more deadly mutated or cancerous cells than normal healthy ones.

This explains why the average person is not born dying of cancer. Because unlike catching a virus, we develop cancer over time through the process of cell degeneration. On the Oprah Winfrey Show, researchers commented about the link between hydrogenated oils and breast cancer. Studies indicate a 40% increase in breast cancer in women eating hydrogenated oils. Now in a normal healthy state, your immune system should have automatically kicked in, and produced the army of white blood cells needed to destroy the mutated cancerous cells. Trans fats lower the body's healthy oxygen-rich, high-alkaline pH into an acidic deadly oxygen deprived condition. All bacteria causing diseases thrive in an environment where oxygen is lacking. This is one of the main reasons why trans fats are equivalent to a hydrogen bomb being dropped inside the human body.

This counterfeit oil literally kills every healthy cell in the body over time through suffocation and structural damage. Unfortunately, our immune systems don't work our entire lives because everyday, were loading our bodies with immune-suppressing refined sugar, cancer-causing artificial sweeteners, and poisonous mineral-depleted table salt. Most of our foods are nutritionally depleted or totally over cooked, and we don't take any kind of herbal remedies or supplements to rectify the problem. Cancerous cells continue growing unabated until they take over and destroy our very lives.

Anyone who eats trans-fats is actually committing nutritional suicide by putting more hydrogen into the body than was ever meant to be present at one time. If you're feeding this hazardous waste material to family and church members, relatives and friends, you're killing them as well. John 10:10 says, "The thief cometh not, but for to steal, and to kill, and to destroy, I am come that they might have life, and that they might have it more abundantly." The hidden trans fatty acids in McDonald's, Hardee's and Arby's french fries cause twice the damage done by regular saturated fats. The fries at Burger King and Wendy's are even worse. There is a two-day supply of artery-clogging trans-fatty acids in many of the meals served at Red Lobster. Those who love Kentucky Fried Chicken can eat a full day's worth of this poison in just one meal. Eating just one Dunkin Donut Old Fashioned Cake donut is equivalent to eating eight strips of bacon in regards to the amount of damage occurring to the arteries due to trans-fatty acids. Innocent looking canned soups that sit on supermarket shelves and are promoted as being good for your health are loaded with hydrogenated oils. There have been recent news report linking McDonald's french fries to breast cancer in women.

A majority of health food and especially junk food snacks also contain trans-fatty acids, so read the labels carefully. Most European countries allow only 4% of trans fatty acids in all foods that are made using hydrogenated oils. Some countries, including Denmark, have outlawed hydrogenated oils for the past 40 years. Intriguingly Denmark has the lowest diagnosed incidents of heart disease, obesity, cancers, diabetes, breast cancer, autoimmune diseases, and other degenerative diseases than any other civilized country in the entire world. What is even more intriguing is that the majority of the fat in their diets is saturated fat from dairy products. Recent studies show that as little as 4% of these trans-fatty acids can cause these diseases to develop.

I guess in the end the real question should be have the minds of humans been able to surpass the mind of God? Has mankind successfully and effectively reversed the divine plan of God by shortening the amount of time that humans live in sin? With all of the scientific and medical research available today, it appears as if mankind has gone overboard in attempting to make humans live longer in their iniquities. In fact, people are suffering and dying prematurely in record numbers so much so that if things aren't reversed, there will be no one left when Christ returns. Can you see how Satan is deceptively trying to make the earth become void of human life. We have commercials with the likes of B.B. king discussing diabetes testing with a young teenager. When I was a child, the only people who got diabetes were older people. Someone having diabetes in their teens was unheard of. Today, elementary children carry to school diabetic testing kits in their lunch sacks. What in the world have we done. These children are supposed to be our future; that's if they ever make it.

The days of blessing and eating oxygen-depleting, cell-deteriorating diseases causing margarine and trans-fatty oils are over! Blessing this garbage will not reverse its catastrophic affects on the human body. You can bless this junk until Christ returns, and the only difference will be is that you'll be saying grace with diabetes, heart disease, cancer, obesity, arthritis and lupus, or a whole host of other degenerative diseases that are ravaging this country today. Again, it is and always has been, about making the right choices. Can we live without trans fats or foods containing hydrogenated oils? Of course we can. Humans had survived for almost 4,400 years before their introduction into the food supply. So it is pretty safe to assume that we can last another 5000 years or until Christ returns. The decision to make is yours, and I hope and pray that after reading this book, you will make the necessary changes and remove this hydrogen bomb from your normal diet. If you don't have the moral strength nor intestinal fortitude to do it for yourself, at least do it for the sake of your children and other loved ones.

There are other oils I recommend in place of trans fatty oils. They include first cold pressed, extra virgin olive oil, peanut oil, coconut oil, and Smart Balance oil or buttery spread. I personally use extra virgin olive oil exclusively and occasionally Smart Balance if I run out of olive oil. Also, evidence concerning flaxseed oil in the diet revealed that it reduces tumors by up to 50%. Your body needs fats to maintain optimum health and function. It's important to supply the temple of God with the right kinds of fats. **Remember, God has placed before you life and death, sickness and disease, so choose life, that you and your seed may live.**

C H A P T E R 6

Health Begins with a Balanced pH

"I have set before you life and death, blessing and cursing: therefore choose life, that both thou and thy seed may live:" (Deuteronomy 30:19)

For most of our lives, we have all been told how vitally important it is to maintain a healthy immune system. We were told that this is the only way to prevent the attacks of viruses and disease from taking over our bodies. We were taught that our body's very first line of defense against any illness is a properly functioning immune system. If our bodies are unable to overcome the symptoms of an impending illness, it's because we have a compromised immune response. In reality, the body's immune system is a secondary response to an internal out of balance pH condition taking place in the blood. I want to point out here that there is a big difference between infectious diseases that are normally caused by viruses or bacterial infections, and degenerative diseases, which are the direct result of unhealthy lifestyle habits. We catch infectious diseases in the same way a wide receiver catches a football. They are passed to us through various modes, the most common being airborne. On the other hand, degenerative diseases like diabetes, heart diseases, obesity, cancer, kidney failure and hypertension develop overtime, and are not passed along to us through the air or in the water.

Most people don't die from catching a cold or flu;, they normally recover as the virus cycles it way out the body. However, millions of people die from degenerative diseases every year, and these diseases are only healed through proper healthy lifestyle habits. The good news is that all degenerative diseases are reversible, if properly treated. Some are healed in as little as a few weeks while others can take several months. It all depends on what goes into the body to keep the blood clean and healthy. Complete and total healing of all degenerative diseases will only take place when and if the condition of the blood is restored to a normal, life-preserving pH balance. This is such a lifesaving statement that I am compelled to repeat it because it cannot be stressed enough. Complete and total healing of all degenerative diseases will only take place when and if the condition of the blood is restored to a normal, life-preserving pH balance. Leviticus 17:11 says, "For the life of the flesh is in the blood." The condition of our health, good or bad, is determined by the state of our blood. Satan wants to defile your blood in the same way that he defiled the earth before God restored order again, Genesis Chapter 1:3, "And God said let there be light."

Your bloodstream is a moving current of life nourishing all of your cells, while at the same time performing the task of waste management by removing deadly toxic materials from the body. To accomplish these vital functions for human survival, it must remain free flowing and unimpeded as it travels throughout the body. Imagine a sweeping vigorous river that flows into brooks and brooks that feed into small streams that nourish the ecosystem. This is how blood should flow through your arteries, from there into your veins, and then diverted into small capillaries that bring sustaining nutrients to every living cell.

A healthy and balanced pH condition leads to healthy organs, which then lead to an invigorating immune system, that is then able to fight and protect against infectious diseases. This explains how the thieves caught during the outbreak of the bubonic plague were able to remain healthy and active in their profession, while millions of other people died all around them. The garlic they ingested enhanced their immune system by first improving the condition of their blood stream. Fresh cut organic garlic produces over 1000 sulfites that destroy bacteria, viruses, parasites, and yeast on contact. The vile odor in garlic forces the liver to contract, releasing bile into the blood to cleanse it. Today, the average person, due to unhealthy lifestyle practices, are walking around with stagnant, congested, and diseased infested currents of death flowing throughout their bodies the majority of their lives. Not only are their internal organs diseased and degenerated, they don't have a healthy immune system to combat attacks on the body. You talk to these types of people all the time who are always sick or complaining about something being wrong with them.

Everything we consume is dead and full of artificial sweeteners which are highly acidic, and depress the body's ability to produce energy. A common every day American meal consists of cooked deal animal flesh, with cooked dead starches, combined with overcooked dead vegetables, and a piece of baked dead bread. This is topped off with some type of highly toxic drink sweetened with sugar or an artificial sweetener. This is just one of the standard meals we consume in this country at least once or twice a day. There is nothing in this meal that is life giving or preserving. This type of typical meal is highly acidic, and actually poisons the blood depleting it of oxygen. You must understand this undeniable fact, *death cannot feed you life*, it can only feed you death. It never has and it never will. This is why things are buried when they die. If death was able to give us life, we would continue using it. Christ was buried, but He also rose again, and it is the fact that He rose again which is most important. Had He simply stayed in the ground, the whole experience of the cross would have been just another crucifixion. No matter how many chemicals you add to death to make it taste mouth watering and smell heavenly, it is still death.

This is the death that flows through your blood everyday, carrying disease and dangerous bacteria to every cell it ultimately ends up feeding. In the simplest terms, we are poisoning ourselves, resulting in unnecessary debilitating sicknesses and premature death, while at the same time, we're trying to maintain a life of vibrancy and optimum health. Instead, we have no energy most of the time, and are always suffering with some type of sickness that occurs monthly or yearly. As a matter of fact, some people actually anticipate getting sick every year during certain seasons. How absurd is this, to actually plan on becoming sick every year. Some people carry around excess weight that becomes impossible to manage as a symptom of the death that they consume, which starts to wear out their vital organs.

The heart, liver, lungs, kidneys, etc. are constantly battling to deal with this toxic environment they are forced to work in, because they're submerged and surrounded by death 24 hours a day. Imagine how effectively you would be able to work if you were surrounded by death everyday, 24 hours a day, 365 days a year, for several decades. At some point, this unhealthy environment would start to take its toll on your health too. This is exactly what every one of our cells experience as they are entombed inside of our bodies. If this cellular situation is not properly resolved first, then the process of metabolic diseases will begin to cripple the body's vital organs, which will then spread and incapacitate your immune and endocrine systems. One will never be able to prevent sickness at the symptom level unless their immune system is functioning at peak performance. In like manner, one cannot stop dysfunctions at the immune level unless the organs that supply the immune system are properly functioning. All of these processes start with the cellular condition of the pH levels in the bloodstream.

What is the pH, and how does it work? pH stands for potential hydrogen and is the measurement of hydrogen ions present in the blood. Increased hydrogen ions result in a drop in the pH which is acidic and oxygen depleting, while a decrease results in a pH rise which is alkaline and oxygen rich. Your car battery contains acid which is fast burning to start your car quickly on cold mornings. The batteries in your flashlight are alkaline which are slow burning to give off light over a long period of time. The Bible teaches that the life of the flesh is in the blood. Refined sugar is highly acidic, which means it burns fast and heats up the blood. This explains why when children are given candy, they can't be still because their cells are burning within the blood. They are actually burning from the inside out, so they hop around as any normal person would and can't be still.

The scale that is used for measuring the pH is from 0 to 14, with 7 being the neutral point. Above 7 is alkaline and below 7 is acidic. The optimal pH of the blood and urine is 7.4, slightly alkaline. The body's pH is directly affected by the various categories of food that are eaten and how well they are broken down. Acidic conditions cause decay through oxidation which can result in the following symptoms: weakening of the skin, hair, nails, teeth, and bones; deterioration of the digestive tract; leaky gut syndrome; candida allergies; excitability of the nervous system; sciatica; feelings of depressive illnesses; anxiety; panic disorders; muscular spasms and cramps; enhanced susceptibility to bacterial and viral infections; chronic fatigue; blockage of certain minerals which become unavailable; and increased risk of cancerous cells proliferating and spreading unabated.

Bacteria and viruses cannot live in an oxygen-rich alkaline environment.

When the pH is kept slightly alkaline at 7.4, the cells have more protection against disease. For example, the egg white of a free range chicken has a highly alkaline pH of 9, while the yolk itself has a slightly acidic pH of 6.5. The egg white with its high alkaline pH protects the yolk from bacteria, fungi, and viruses. This environment remains slightly alkaline while life is forming and developing with the millions of cells forming the new chicken. The cells within our body need this same type of balanced matrix as they die off and new cells are reborn. Hydrogen is composed of two words: hydro, meaning water, and gen which is from the Greek meaning genes. So hydrogen means "born of water" and reflects the birthing process of most species. Our bodies are comprised of 75% water (H_2O), which means that there are two hydrogen atoms surrounding one oxygen atom in each molecule of water.

The word oxygen is also divided into two words: oxy, meaning acid or combustible, and gen which again comes from the Greek word genes meaning born. So we can interpret oxygen as the "burning of new genes." Hence, new life is protected as it forms within this divinely balanced matrix. Does this not mirror our spiritual regeneration, as we are born again into new creatures through the baptism of water and fire. We become new spiritual creatures in Christ by means of this perfectly balanced ordained spiritual matrix. All cell regeneration must maintain this divine symmetry or disease and deformities will occur.

The following factors will have an influence on the pH level of the body. Acidic foods such as fast foods, meats, processed grains, some fruits like ripe bananas and plums, refined salt, sugar, condiments, pickles, ketchup, soda pop, and almost all refined, processed foods, etc. have a pH ranging from 2.8 to 5.5 which is highly acidic. These types of foods, including the consumption of excess meat, tear down our health. Healing foods that restore health include: almonds, unpasteurized honey, bee pollen, maple syrup, figs, dates, raw organic yogurt and cheese, earth/root vegetables, green vegetables, apricots, avocados, coconut, grapes, molasses, raisins, and lemons. These are all alkaline-forming foods.

Your thoughts and emotions can also greatly affect the condition of your blood. Emotions of happiness, joy, and love tend to create alkaline-forming chemical reactions in the body. However, the opposite emotions of anger, fear, jealousy, and hate create acidic-forming chemical reactions in the body. Processed foods as a whole are highly acidic and promote premature death. Junk food is the worst and is probably why it is called junk food. Distilled water sprinkled with Celtic Sea Salt promotes wellness and fights against cancer.

Thus, natural sea salt can also help in correcting excess acidity, restoring good digestion, relieving allergies and skin diseases, removing excess acids surrounding the brain, and preventing many forms of cancer. This natural salt provides a steady boost in cellular energy and gives the body a heightened resistance to infections and bacterial diseases. The following alkaline forming foods should be eaten on a regular basis: apricots, molasses, cucumbers, avocados, lemons, coconut, all melons, figs, dates, raisins, organic yogurt, grapes, unpasteurized honey, maple syrup, root vegetables, alfalfa and bean sprouts, cayenne pepper, algae, Chlorella, with the best alkalizing food being raw untreated almonds. Soaking the almonds for 24 hours prior to consumption starts the germination process in the seed and thus activates its life force. Eating almonds for breakfast is a good way to start the morning. Most commercial flours as with all junk foods are highly acidic. I recommend that everyone bake their own bread, pastries, and cakes.

When the body is acidic, its ability to absorb minerals and nutrients is greatly diminished. This also decreases the energy production in cells, their ability to repair damaged cells, and detoxify heavy metals. Unfortunately, it also allows tumor cells to thrive, and makes us more susceptible to fatigue and afflictions. Because the typical American diet consists of far too many acidic producing foods, acidosis is more common in our society. We simply consume far too much meat, eggs, dairy, refined products, coffee and pop, and not enough alkaline producing fresh vegetables and fruits. We use too many drugs which are acid forming, and we use artificial chemical sweeteners like Splenda, Sweet 'N Low, NutraSweet, and Equal, or generically Aspartame, which are poisons and extremely acid forming. One of the best things we can do to correct an overly acid body is to clean up the diet and lifestyle. To maintain health, the diet should consist of 60% alkaline forming foods and 40% acid forming foods.

To restore health, the diet should consist of 80% alkaline forming foods and 20% acid forming foods. Generally, alkaline forming foods include: most fruits, green vegetables, peas, beans, lentils, spices, herbal seasonings, and seeds and nuts.

Alkalizing Vegetables

Alfalfa, Barley Grass, Beet Greens, Beets, Broccoli, Cabbage, Carrot, Cauliflower, Celery, Chard Greens, Chlorella, Collard Greens, Cucumber, Dandelions, Dulce, Edible Flowers, Eggplant, Fermented Veggies, Garlic,Green Beans, Green Peas, Kale, Kohlrabi, Lettuce,

Alkalizing Vegetables (continued)

Mushrooms, Mustard Greens, Nightshade Veggies, Onions, Parsnips (high glycemic), Peas, Peppers, Pumpkin, Radishes, Rutabaga, Sea Veggies, Spinach, Green Spirulina, Sprouts, Sweet Potatoes, Tomatoes, Watercress, Wheat Grass, Wild Greens

Alkalizing Oriental Vegetables

Daikon, Dandelion Root, Kombu, Maitake, Nori, Reishi, Shitake, Umeboshi,Wakame.

Alkalizing Fruits

Apple, Apricot, Avocado, Berries, Blackberries, Cantaloupe, Cherries, Coconut, Fresh Currants, Dates, Dried Figs, Dried Grapes, Grapefruit, Honeydew Melon, Lemon, Lime, Muskmelons, Nectarine, Orange, Peach, Pear, Pineapple, Raisins, Raspberries, Rhubarb, Strawberries, Tangerine, Tomato, Tropical Fruits, Umeboshi Plums, Watermelon

Alkalizing Protein

Almonds (raw), Chestnuts, Millet, Tempeh (fermented), Tofu (fermented), Whey Protein Powder, Eggs (poached), Cottage Cheese, Chicken Breast, Yogurt, Chestnuts, Flax Seeds, Pumpkin Seeds, Squash Seeds, Sunflower Seeds, Millet, Sprouted Seeds, Nuts.

Alkalizing Sweeteners

Stevia: 100 times sweeter than sugar, very bitter use sparingly.

Alkalizing Spices & Seasonings

Chili Pepper, Cinnamon, Curry, Ginger, Herbs (all), Miso, Mustard, Sea Salt, Tamari.

Alkalizing Other

Alkaline Antioxidant Water, Apple Cider Vinegar, Bee Pollen, Fresh Fruit Juice, Green Juices, Lecithin Granules, Mineral Water, Blackstrap Molasses, Probiotic Cultures, Soured Dairy Products (organic yogurt, buttermilk, etc.) Veggie Juices, Chlorella, Green Tea, Herbal Tea, Dandelion Tea, Ginseng Tea, Banchi Tea, Kombucha.

Alkalizing Minerals

Calcium: pH 12, Cesium: pH 14, Magnesium: pH 9, Potassium: pH 14, Sodium: pH 14,

Although it might seem that citrus fruits would have an acidifying effect on the body, the citric acid they contain actually has an alkalinizing effect in the system. Note that a food's acid or alkaline forming tendency in the body has nothing to do with the actual pH of the food itself. For example, lemons are very acidic; however, the end products they produce after digestion and assimilation are very alkaline, so lemons are alkaline forming in the body. Likewise, meat will test alkaline before digestion, but it leaves very acidic residue in the body. Like nearly all animal products, meat is very acid forming.

Acidifying Vegetables

Corn, Lentils, Olives, Winter Squash

Acidifying Fruits

Blueberries, Canned or Glazed Fruits, Cranberries, Currants, Plums, Ripe Bananas

Acidifying Grains

Amaranth, Barley, Bran, Oat Bran, Wheat Bread, Corn, Cornstarch, Crackers, Soda, Flour, Wheat Flour, White Hemp Seed Flour, Kamut, Macaroni, Noodles, Oatmeal, Oats (rolled), Quinoa, Rice (all), Rice Cakes, Rye, Spaghetti, Spelt, Wheat Germ, Wheat

Acidifying Beans & Legumes

Almond Milk, Black Beans, Chick Peas, Green Peas, Kidney Beans, Lentils, Pinto Beans, Red Beans, Rice Milk, Soy Beans, Soy Milk, White Beans

Acidifying Dairy

Butter, Cheese, Processed, Ice Cream, Ice Milk

Acidifying Nuts & Butters
Cashews, Legumes, Peanut Butter, Peanuts, Pecans, Tahini, Walnuts

Acidifying Animal Protein
Bacon, Beef, Carp, Clams, Cod, Corned Beef, Fish, Haddock, Lamb, Lobster, Mussels, Organ Meats, Oyster, Pike, Pork, Rabbit, Salmon, Sardines, Sausage, Scallops, Shellfish, Shrimp, Tuna, Turkey, Veal, Venison

Acidifying Fats & Oils
Avocado Oil, Butter, Canola Oil, Corn Oil, Flax Oil, Hemp Seed Oil, Lard, Olive Oil, Safflower Oil, Sesame Oil, Sunflower Oil

Acidifying Sweeteners
Carob, Corn Syrup, Refined Sugar, Artificial Sweeteners (Aspartame, saccharin, Splenda, etc.)

Acidifying Other Foods
Catsup, Cocoa, Coffee, Mustard, Pepper, Soft Drinks, Vinegar

Acidifying Drugs and Chemicals
Aspirin, Chemicals, Drugs, Medicinal (all pharmaceuticals - prescription or over the counter), Drugs, Psychedelic Herbicides, Pesticides, Tobacco

ALKALINE: Love, joy, peace, patience, kindness, goodness, faithfulness, gentleness and self control. Fruits of the Spirit that preserve life and against such things there is no law.

ACIDIC: Hatred, discord, jealousy, fits of rage, envy, drunkenness. Sinful nature destroying life and shall not inherit the kingdom of God. The intended purpose of both the "Daily Nutritional Regimen" and the "Daily Meal Planner" is to help educate you on the best way to prevent and reverse existing degenerative diseases, help rebuild the body's immune system, balance the pH of all bodily fluids, help with permanent weight loss and weight management, reduce and eliminate the need for prescription medications, and to bring overall balance and healing to the entire person.

Daily Nutritional Regimen
Warning: Avoid all products that contain aluminum and trans-fatty

oils or hydrogenated or partially hydrogenated oils (this includes margarine) and other products containing this poison. Be careful of products that say 0 trans fats, but yet contain hydrogenated oils. These ingredients are linked to Alzheimer's, brain tumors, diabetes, heart disease, obesity, several forms of cancer including breast cancer, and hypertension. They are highly acidic in the blood causing oxygen depravation, cell deformities, and inhibit the ability of cells to function properly.

All Items Should be Organic Whenever Possible

Remember all proteins and starches must be eaten separately.

Foods to Limit and Avoid

Avoid: seafood and pork, non-scaled fish, processed meats, (non-oraganic) canned foods, commercially processed milk and dairy products to include cheese, refined sugar and artificial sweeteners, table salt and salt seasonings, white flour, bleached wheat products, fried foods, soft drinks and coffee, whole eggs, white rice, roasted nuts, salad dressings, processed foods, junk foods, hydrogenated oils.

Limit: meat consumption of all kinds, fish is okay in moderation; this is where some organic dairy products are okay excluding milk; fruit juices are okay if you are juicing at home. In such cases, drink as much as you want. Limit also whole wheat products like pastas and bread.

Sweeteners: all refined sugar and artificial sweeteners should be immediately replaced with stevia, maple syrup, honey, blackstrap molasses, or turbinado (raw sugar).

Seasoning Salts: all seasoning salts and table salt should be discarded and replaced with Celtic Sea Salt.

Herbal Seasonings: use non-irradiated herbs as much as possible.

It is very important that you do not overcook your meals. The following items should be consumed **raw** on a daily basis: garlic, onions, raw fruits, raw vegetables, organic ground flaxseed, first cold press extra virgin olive oil, raw nuts (¼ to ½ cup of the following daily: sunflower seeds, almonds, pumpkin seeds, walnuts, cashews, pecans, hazelnuts sprinkled with Celtic Sea Salt and coated with olive oil; can be eaten as a snack, sprinkled on top of a salad, or with a meal in place of chicken, fish, turkey and other meats), whole grains, lentils, oats, beans, etc.

Daily Detox: ½ lemon, 8 oz. cup of distilled water, cayenne pepper (½ teaspoon), maple syrup or stevia, and a pinch of Celtic Sea Salt.

Breakfast: organic cereals, oatmeal, fruits, flaxseed, wheat germ, oat bran, sesame seed, rice milk, maple syrup, whole home baked wheat toast, pancakes, waffles, bagels (no cream cheese). Cereals should contain no refined sugar or artificial sweeteners. Diabetics should use soy milk instead of rice milk for cereals. Oatmeal can be sweetened with 100% maple syrup, stevia, raisins, or all natural apple sauce. Ground flaxseed and wheat germ can be sprinkled over cereals, fresh fruit, salads, and mixed into a glass of water or juice.

Lunch: salads, beans, fish, (chicken and turkey should be boiled and then baked afterward; simply brush olive oil onto boiled meats and poultry along with pepper and sodium-free herbal seasonings. After baking, sprinkle on Celtic Sea Salt moderately and enjoy.), vegetables of all types. Drink only distilled water with meal if you must have water. Sprinkle Celtic Sea salt moderately over all your foods.

Dinner: eat a plethora of mixed vegetables, seeds, nuts, ground flax-seed, egg whites only, whole wheat bread. Meal should be 70% raw and 30% cooked. A small amount of rice or whole wheat pasta is okay.

Snack: fruits, nuts and seeds, or drink fruit juices between meals

These are perfectly balanced meals which will heal the body from the inside out. Weight loss will naturally become manageable. Remember, if you are taking prescription drugs or have fatty liver syndrome, you will have a much more difficult time losing and managing your weight.

Daily Meal Planner

The purpose of this plan is to teach you how to eat foods in their proper combinations and timing. This will ensure proper digestion, assimilation, and removal of waste. No longer will you eat and feel sluggish and tired afterwards, but energetic and alert. More importantly, you will reduce parasitic, bacterial, fungal, and mold infestations, because there will be no food spoiling and fermenting in your intestines.

Important Notes:

1) Start each morning with 22-28 ounces of warm water.

2) Do not drink any fluids with your meals unless you must. Drink liquids between meals. Try to do your own juicing; avoid soft drinks and coffee. Your drink of choice should be distilled water. **3)** If you are short on time, you can prepare your cooked portions in advance and refrigerate them. **4)** You can always change the order of these meals at your discretion. **5)** Between meals you can munch on raw nuts in moderation and fruits, vegetables, or fruit juices. Try to avoid all processed snack foods and dairy products. If you must eat them, be sure to drink lots of distilled water with fresh squeezed lemon.

Monday

Breakfast: Start with fresh fruit such as melons, apples, grapes, peaches, etc. All fruits in this group should be non-acidic like grapefruit, kiwi, oranges, etc. Wait 20 minutes after eating fruits before continuing breakfast. Whole organic oats, Cream of Wheat, organic grits, dry cereals, soy milk (for diabetics) or rice milk.

Lunch: Organic spring salad, topped with chicken or nuts or beans, and a side dish of vegetables. Salad dressing(½ squeezed lemon, 2 Tbsp. olive oil, 1 tsp. apple cider vinegar, 8oz. distilled water, Celtic Sea Salt, pepper, and non-irradiated herbal seasonings); shake well.

Dinner: Vegetable medley, whole wheat bread, small portion of steamed brown rice or whole wheat pasta, boiled or baked potatoes.

Tuesday

Breakfast: Start with fresh fruit (melons, apples, grapes, peaches, etc.). Follow same as Monday or have organic whole wheat pancakes, waffles, or ½ cup almonds.

Lunch: Fish, small with scales only like salmon, Tilapia, bass, perch, whiting. Fish should be organically raised. Can be baked or broiled, served with salad and mixed vegetables.

Tuesday

Dinner: baked potato, mixed vegetables, salad, whole wheat bread.

Wednesday (continued)

Breakfast: start with fresh fruit (melons, apples, grapes, peaches, etc.). Follow same as Monday or have organic homemade yogurt.

Lunch: Lamb chops or chicken (baked or broiled). Serve with salad and mixed vegetables.

Dinner: Wheat pasta served with sauteed cabbage and sun dried tomatoes, mixed vegetables, salad, whole wheat bread.

Thursday

Breakfast: Start with fresh fruit (melons, apples, grapes, peaches, etc.). All fruits in this group should be non-acidic like grapefruit, kiwi, oranges, etc.. Wait 20 minutes after eating fruits before continuing breakfast. Whole organic oats, Cream of Wheat, organic grits, dry cereals, with soy milk (for diabetics) or rice milk.

Lunch: organic spring salad topped with cashews, almonds, sunflower seeds, and pumpkin seeds. Mixed vegetables.

Dinner: Steamed brown rice, mixed vegetables, salad, whole wheat bread.

Friday

Breakfast: Start with fresh fruit (melons, apples, grapes, peaches, etc.). All fruits in this group should be non-acidic like grapefruit, kiwi, oranges, etc.. Wait 20 minutes after eating fruits before continuing breakfast. Organic whole wheat pancakes, waffles, or ½ cup almonds.

Lunch: Organic spring salad, topped with tofu or nuts, or beans, and a side dish of vegetables. Salad dressing (½ squeezed lemon, 2 Tbsp. olive oil, 1 tsp. apple cider vinegar, 8oz. distilled water, Celtic Sea Salt, pepper, and non-irradiated herbal seasonings); shake well.

Friday (continued)

> **Dinner**: baked potato, mixed vegetables, salad, whole wheat bread

Saturday

> **Breakfast**: Start with fresh fruit (melons, apples, grapes, peaches, etc.) All fruits in this group should be non-acidic like grapefruit, kiwi, oranges, etc. Wait 20 minutes after eating fruits before continuing breakfast. Organic whole wheat pancakes, waffles, or ½ cup almonds.

> **Lunch:** Fish, small with scales only like salmon, Tilapia, bass, perch, whiting. Fish should be organically raised. Can be baked or broiled; serve with salad and mixed vegetables.

> **Dinner:** Wheat pasta served with sauteed cabbage and sun dried tomatoes, mixed vegetables, salad, whole wheat bread.

Sunday

> This is your free day. Eat whatever you want. Remember to drink a tall glass of distilled water and lemon with every meal and all throughout the day.

This meal plan includes meats only as way to eventually wean yourself off of them instead of trying to quit cold turkey.

In a perfect world, humans should be able to handle the symptoms of an oncoming sickness before it becomes full blown. The body should always be on the defense, searching for foreign invaders who look to take over. When these invaders are isolated, they should be properly dealt with and passed out of the body. After the attack is adverted, the body sends out an army of doctor cells to restore order and repair any damages caused by the foreign invaders. They carry calcium directly to the injury and initiate the healing process. This process is impossible without the constant replenishing of properly balanced minerals. Despite our physical differences and make up, the one common bond that we all share is degenerative diseases. It doesn't matter what color or race you are. No ethnicity is spared when it comes to metabolic degenerative disease.

Presently, there are over 300 million people around the world suffering with diabetes and obesity, which is expected to shorten life expectancy by five to nine years. Young and old, male and female, no one is immune to the insidious damages caused by degenerative diseases. Even infants are being born today with diabetes, having to take medication before getting the bottle. This is why it is so important to maintain proper cellular health first. If the cellular integrity remains intact, then the organs of the body will function properly. This will lead to a vibrant immune and endocrine system. All life begins with tiny microscopic cells, and the human body is comprised of over 80 trillion of them that automatically regenerate every second of your life. This is the magnanimity of God's grace in that 1) He has assured that we have more than enough cells, and 2) cell regeneration is perpetual and totally independent of human influence or effort. So it doesn't matter if you are asleep, drunk, or drugged up. God has designed it so that our bodies don't have to totally depend on us for its own survival. If this were the case, many of us would be in a lot of trouble because we'd forget to breathe, swallow, or grow new skin and hair cells.

In a normally healthy body, harmless bacteria called microzymas safely perform evolved aerobic fermentation, as seen when fruits ferment into wine, or the healthy bacteria that grows in the gut wall like acidophilus, plantarum, lactobacillus, etc. However when the blood remains in a an acidic, oxygen-deprived condition for too long, the cells become loaded with toxic waste and start dying off prematurely. This sends a signal to the healthy microzymas to return organisms back to the soil. This bacteria now goes through a process call pleomorphism which means to change to many forms. These new forms are microscopic yeast, molds, viruses, and other microforms that act as a clean-up crew eating away at dead cells and tissue. It is the perpetual microzymas that causes a dead animal to decompose back to soil, returning life back to the dust of the earth from where it came.

Cells are the bricks and mortar from which all living tissue and organs are made. More than 90 nutrients from nine different categories are necessary ingredients for proper cell regeneration and function. When all of these ingredients are present, the body can produce proteins, hormones, etc. If more than half of the more than 90 nutrients are missing, the cells' manufacturing potential is cut in half. Think for a moment if your paycheck was reduced by half. Your buying potential would be greatly impacted. With missing nutrients, our cells have limited energy production, which then limits performance of the entire body. God's mission is to replenish the earth and make it habitable with His image and likeness to preserve His creation. Satan's mission is to un-inhabit the earth with anything that resembles God or his creativity. God's commandment to mankind was to be fruitful (alkaline/ righteous). Satan wants us to be unfruitful (acidic/unrighteous), to make the earth violent and uninhabitable. He wants to deceive you into believing that demons are in control in stead of you knowing the truth about what's lacking inside your body. The counterfeit and the truth are at work in full affect.

Look at how many believers are loading themselves and their children up with oxygen-depriving refined sugar and then going on a diet, both of which are not mentioned in the Bible. It appears as though they have taken the bait, and thus are being destroyed in direct proportions as non-believers, suffering with the same degenerative afflictions. Elderly believers are having to come out of retirement and depend on friends and family, because prescription drug costs are sending them into poverty. How can you talk about delivering anybody else if you are unable to deliver yourself. Believers are putting their trust in heart defibrillators, which manufacturers have just had the largest recall in the history of this country. Many of these devices have started to malfunction, with some people actually dying. Doctors have outsmarted themselves, and can't figure out how to fix this problem before more deaths occur.

After his resurrection, Jesus taught his disciples for 40 days about being a witnesses for the kingdom of God. He used himself as an example of how believers should live a vivacious, vibrant, and victorious life. He promised to send the Holy Spirit to empower us to be effective witnesses. It is amazing how many believers are professing to be full of the Holy Spirit, yet are powerless when it comes to keeping their temples clean and in proper working order. Listen carefully, poison is poison. If you consume it, you will suffer the consequences. Stop giving the enemy victory over your lives by following his deceptive tactics. He knows exactly what he is doing, and as long as he can keep you believing that dark, unseen spiritual forces are controlling your lives, you and your family will continue taking medications, suffering with afflictions, and dying prematurely. Every minute, a believer dies from heart disease. If God cannot force you to live Holy, then Satan cannot force you to defile the temple. We are simply choosing to put too much of the wrong things into our bodies, and not enough of the right things. **Remember, God has placed before you life and death, sickness and disease, so choose life, that you and your seed may live.**

The Psychological Battles

"I have set before you life and death, blessing and cursing: therefore choose life, that both thou and thy seed may live:" (Deuteronomy 30:19)

Believers and non-believers alike are under attack by the chief antagonist and false accuser of mankind, Satan. This spiritual assault mentioned in Ephesians 6:12 says, "Our struggle is not against flesh and blood, but against the rulers, authorities, and powers of this dark world, and evil forces in the heavenly realms." The enemy has deceived us into believing that we can just bless and eat anything and everything we want, and still maintain a healthy lifestyle. People are blessing and eating their foods everyday, yet they are dying prematurely and suffering with debilitating illnesses like diabetes, cancer, obesity, heart diseases and hypertension. Yes, we attend church faithfully and participate in the worship services. We are praying and seeking out miracles at the alter, yet the majority of the time, our bodies are fully medicated, keeping us functional until our next dosage. It is a never ending evil and vicious cycle of blessing, eating, and medicating; blessing, eating, and medicating; blessing, eating, and medicating.

As you read this book, the Federal Government is looking into 150 price and marketing fraud cases involving more than 500 drugs. One company in particular by the name of Serono, a Swiss pharmaceutical company, recently settled a $704 million lawsuit. The company developed an AIDS drug that wasn't bringing in profits. So in order to boost sales, the company executives started bribing doctors by giving them financial kickbacks and free trips to the coast of France. Just one 12-week treatment of this drug cost a staggering $21,000. The company also conspired to introduce new drugs into the market for AIDS patients that had not been approved by the FDA, nor had it undergone any kind of trial testing for public safety. Here is the most shocking part of this story. The Federal Government has stated that up to 85% of the prescriptions written were totally unnecessary. Look at how far these dark and evil forces who are at work against us will go to try and destroy our lives.

Five former executives of the company were indicted as a result of company employees who turned whistle blowers. This is where the spiritual battle mentioned in Ephesians crosses over into our physical lives. 1st Timothy 6:10 says, "For the love of money is the root of all evil: which while some coveted after, they have erred from the faith, and pierced themselves through with many arrows." By tempting mankind to covet or desire money, Satan seduces them into breaking the law in order to make a dollar. In this particular case, the company made over $300 million through acts of deception and fraud. The spiritual battle now has accomplished two things. It has caused mankind to turn from the faith for worldly gain. Now mankind is further maimed and destroyed through deception and greed. Satan doesn't care how he takes you out, just as long as he takes you out. The executives at Serono put their interest and lust for money ahead of public safety, even at the risk of people needlessly dying. There are thousands of company executives from Enron to World Comm, who have put their pockets first over the pension funds and retirement plans of their employees.

Our adversary is full of wisdom, and he figured out thousands of years ago how to take the battle from his spiritual realm over into our physical world. All he needs is one person who is willing to take the bait for personal gain or profit, and the rest is history. There is an ironic twist to this story. Each one of the four employees who blew the whistle on the company executives received $51 million each as reward money for their testimony. Look how the executives pierced themselves without even realizing what was coming down the road. Look at how the love of money worked both ways, to commit a crime, and also to convict the criminals who committed the crime.

However, let's reflect back on the thousands of people not really in need of costly medications, but were told by their doctors that they were absolutely necessary. These doctors add to the reasons why doctors and hospitals are the number three killer in the country. Thousands of people are maimed and killed every year from wrong prescriptions, medical mis-diagnoses, and unnecessary medical proce-dures. Satan has been at work since the creation of mankind to remove the image and likeness of God from the face of the earth. He is upset because God restored and repopulated the earth that Satan caused to become void. Not only did God restore order to the earth in Genesis, Chapter One, but this time He made sure that he would be represented throughout the world. Now Satan is highly upset, because he hates God, and everywhere he goes throughout the earth, he is surrounded by the image and likeness of God. What really gets him angry is the fact that there is nothing he can do about it. So Satan has been trying to wipe man off the face of the earth ever since Genesis, Chapter One. Since all of his attempts have failed thus far, he has now focused his attention on the future. Knowing that Christ will return and establish his kingdom here on earth, Satan doesn't want there to be anyone living here when He returns, especially believers with any faith. So he has used deception and greed to defile our food supply and medicines. With harmful foods and medications, we poison and toxify our blood, the life of the flesh.

Here is a staggering new statistic. The medical community now states that children who develop diabetes at the ages of 13 to16 will face life threatening complications, to include premature death by the age of 30, from complications associated with diabetes such as heart disease, kidney failure, obesity and hypertension. Diabetes is the number one cause of kidney failure. Once end-stage kidney disease occurs, the risk of death from cardiovascular disease spikes up to 20 times higher according to many studies. Also the same medications used to treat diabetes are the same medications that eventually lead to kidney failure according to researchers.

In just 4400 years, the life span of mankind has gone from a high of 969 years to just 30 to 60 years. What's disheartening about this picture is the fact that the patriarchs lived to reach old age in good health, with Noah bearing children at the age of 500, while we can barely reach into our early thirties without the care of a doctor and prescription medications. If we do happen to make it to the ripe old age of 60, fertility and reproduction makes the headline news. We are not going to live forever, but we should be able to remain healthy until we die. The state of our health and longevity will all be determined by the condition of our blood. In the same way we needed.

the blood of Christ untainted by sin to save us spiritually, we need to keep our blood clean to save our physical lives.

We get excited and shout around the church because we can speak in tongues, lay hands, and out dance everyone around us. When really, we should be shouting and dancing because we no longer need to rely on drugs to treat our diabetes, cancer, hypertension, heart disease, and obesity. We should dance when we don't have to risk our lives while taking arthritis drugs like Vioxx, now known to have killed up to 30,000 people. Or we no longer have to treat our hypertension with drugs that increase our chances of developing diabetes which leads to kidney failure, which leads to heart disease.

We should get excited and shout because we no longer have to take pain medications like Aleve or Tylenol, which increase the risk of both heart attacks and stroke by 50%. Why are we shouting while at the same time, we're poisoning our children with drugs like Ritalin, which the government is now warning causes depression and brain dysfunction. Why are we falling out all over the church and continue transferring the wealth of the righteous out of the kingdom of God? We shouldn't open our mouths, or move our feet, or lay hands on anybody else until our faith stands firm and doubtless in God's abilities to change us first. Instead of trying to deliver other folks, wouldn't it make more sense to ask God's help in delivering us from our unhealthy and even deadly generational habits, habits which have caused us to become afflicted in the first place. Jesus promised not to leave us as orphans, but to send us the Counselor, the Holy Spirit, who would teach us in all things.

Knowing that we are to continue the work of Christ here on the earth in our physical bodies, it would make sense that the Counselor would have something to teach us and say about our physical well being. After all, He has to operate with us until Christ returns; just a thought. If God has ordained what He has placed in the earth to naturally heal our bodies, then we must take him at His word and trust that He can do it. How did the patriarchs live so healthy without medical and scientific advancements. They just stuck to the nutritional plan commanded by God for mankind. Today, we are so far away from the diet God originally gave us, and we can see the results of this all around us. We must return back to the beginning in order to correct our present and future. It works for the animals and it will certainly work for us. We are supposed to be representing the likeness and image of God by being the light and salt of the earth. How will the world be able to see us, if we are dimly lit and under a blanket of sickness and disease, full of mineral-depleted salt which has lost its savor. Mark 9:50 says, "Salt is good, but if the salt loses it flavor, how will you season it? Have salt in yourselves, and have peace with one another."

Jesus says if we've lost our saltiness we cannot preserve peace on the earth. Now if we can't preserve the earth, we are no good to the kingdom of God. You see, throughout the Bible, salt symbolizes the restoration of peace. Every covenant God made and every sacrifice offered to God by the priest was done with an oblation of salt. We are supposed to salt the earth with peace, but it appears as if the church is just as quick tempered as the next person. Salt acts as an antiseptic which slows the growth of micro-organisms. That's why it is used in the packaging of dead animal products you buy in the grocery store. It slows down the progression of decomposing bacteria. A restored covenant relationship with God also acts as an antiseptic, by slowing down the growth of sin in our lives. While neither the covenant nor the salt can totally destroy the sin or micro-organisms, having both of them in our lives can slow their progression, thus enabling us to preserve the earth and live in peace.

It is amazing how everyone seems to have a word from the Lord. Everyone is either a prophet, an apostle, or has some deep spiritual connection with God with so much so-called spiritual revelation and interpretation coming from heaven today. What is the Holy Spirit really saying to the church about how we mistreat the temple that He has to operate through? Remember, the Holy Spirit's role is to continue the work of Christ here on the earth until Christ returns. If He is going to successfully complete this momentous task, He will need properly functioning temples. What is the Spirit saying to the church about our lifestyle that appears to conform to that of the world. We're on the same types of diets, eat the same disease generating foods, and take the same dangerous medications. Romans 12:2 says, "Be not conformed to this world," and yet in ignorance, the church has conformed to this world in almost every area that pertains to our physical bodies. In stubbornness and carelessness, we are now paying an extremely heavy penalty as millions suffer and are afflicted with a record number of infirmities. In fact, we all look pretty much the same. Diabetes, cancer, hypertension, obesity, and heart disease are prevalent both inside and outside the church. Exodus 15:26 says, "If thou wilt diligently hearken to the voice of the Lord thy God and will do that which is right in his sight, and wilt give ear to his commandments, and keep all his statutes, I will put none of the diseases upon thee, which I have brought upon the Egyptians. For I am the Lord who heals you."

How can the Holy Spirit give you a word regarding the welfare of everybody else, but have nothing to say to you about your own. Are we really hearing from the Lord, or are we hearing for ourselves only what we want to hear. There are just too many believers who are sick and debilitated, feeding their families sickness and disease, and having their faith tied to medications to simply be ignored. Too much wealth is yet being transferred from the kingdom of God. We should get excited because our ability to function properly is not hampered by the side affects brought on by so many toxic medications.

Last year, believers spent some $300 billion on health care and not one person was healed. The symptoms were just masked by the medication, as the sickness moved to the next weakest organ in the body. That's why you are warned not to take medications if you have another underlying issue not related to the current issue. As a matter of fact, where are all the so-called healthy people who are recovering and completely off all their medications. Do you know that every time you take an antibiotic, you adversely alter the body's normal healthy flora. If the sick are actually recovering and being cured of their ailments, why are they still taking medications. If you fix a flat tire and then continue to fill it up with air, eventually it will burst. Once the tire is completely repaired, it doesn't need air anymore.

Many of us are getting along just fine spiritually, but physically we are slowly dying and suffering with debilitating illnesses. This style of living seems to greatly contradict 3rd John 1:2 which says, "I pray that you may enjoy good health and that all may go well with you even as your soul is getting along well. 1st Corinthians 6:19 says"Your body is the temple of the Holy Spirit who is in you, whom you have received from God. You are not your own. 20) You were bought at a price; therefore, honor God with your body. Isn't it amazing to think that the same foods we are told to eat as children, we are told to start avoiding as we get older. Song of Solomon 3:15 speaks of the little foxes that destroy the vine or body. Back in biblical days, farmers would grow grape orchards on their land. At night, foxes would come around and eat any loose chickens that were not locked away. However, if there were no loose chickens around, the foxes would go over to the grape orchard and eat the grapes. The baby foxes were too short and couldn't reach up to the grapes, so they would nibble at the vine.

This constant nibbling on the vine or body over time would eventually destroy the entire orchard. So it is with our bodies. The constant nibbling on foods that have been stripped of all nutritional value, then polluted with all kinds of toxic chemicals, additives, salt which has lost its savor, drug-addicting sugar, and preservatives that were never meant to enter our bodies, simply poisons and destroys us over time. Satan doesn't have to fight God over us. We make his job easy by slowly destroying the vine, the body, the temple, and ourselves.

I come from a very large family of 24 aunts and uncles and unfortunately, I've been to more funerals than birthday parties. The majority of the causes of death were either cancer or heart disease. It is interesting to note the fact that none of my aunts or uncles were born with any of the diseases they eventually died from. They didn't catch cancer or heart disease by simply sitting next to a contagious person infected with these disease. If that were possible, we would all be in big trouble. Since these diseases were not passed through the process of viral or bacterial infection (their outer environment), their internal environment is the only other possible answer. These diseases all developed over time from a lifetime of acidic-producing nutrition and lack of proper hydration. There are thousands of highly toxic, acid producing preservatives and chemical additives used in the processing of our foods today. Yet, only a third of them are deemed to be safe by the Food and Drug Administration.

Add up all of the preservatives, food colorings, additives and chemicals, in addition to the drug-addicting refined sugar and deadly mineral-depleted salts that we feed to our children. What happens? Their little bodies go into immediate toxic shock. You think your child is demon possessed? No! They are full of unclean foods and poisons, and lack the proper balance of minerals a healthy body requires to function properly. Parents are medicating their children with drugs like Ritalin just to help alter and calm their behavior. There are just as many drug addicts in the church as there are outside the church. If you were to add up all of the people in the church who are addicted to sugar and caffeine, then add to this list all those who are taking prescription medications and over-the-counter drugs, you'll end up with a staggering number of addicted church goers.

This is why, as believers, it is so important not to pass judgment on the habits of other people, because in the same way you judge their addictions, you are just as guilty in your own. Just because it's sugar instead of crack cocain or heroin you are addicted to doesn't make it any better. Both defile the temple and both will eventually lead to sickness and death. By the way, sugar and heroin are both made through similar processes. Both are highly addictive and habit forming. My friend, there is no magic pill or cure. The only true cure is the Gospel. 1st Peter 1:16 says, "Be Holy, because I am holy." John 10:10 says, "The thief comes only but to steal, kill, and destroy." He comes trying to steal your eternal inheritance, kill the temple where the Holy Spirit dwells, and to destroy your faith. Remember, without faith it is impossible to please God.

Satan understands that there are many believers who have a form of Godliness but deny the power thereof. He truly understands the importance of faith as it relates to the life of all believers and their personal relationship with God. Hebrew 11:6 says, "But without faith it is impossible to please Him, for he that cometh to God must believe that He is, and that He is a rewarder of them that diligently seek Him." Many people believe in God, but not in His power or abilities. In Luke18:8, Jesus asked a disheartening question to His disciples, "Nevertheless, when the Son of Man comes, will He really find faith in the earth?" In other words, after all that I have gone through already-- my death and resurrection, the pain, suffering, and humiliation I've already endured, the many miracles I performed to increase mans' faith in Me-- with all that I've accomplished, will it be enough to keep faith here in the earth until I return?

Jesus asked as if He already knew the answer to this question. You see, pain can cause a person to lose their enthusiasm rather quickly, and it appears as though believers use just as many prescription medications as non-believers. I hate to say this, but today many people have more faith in their little pill bottle than the Word of God. Sadly I ask, will Jesus really find faith in the earth upon His return? It appears that the animals who are under our dominion trust God more than we do, for you see when they get sick, they will instinctively eat on grass and leaves. Genesis 1:29 gave us every seed bearing herb for food, and Revelation 22:2 says that the leaves shall be for the healing of the nations. It appears as though we've got it all mixed up.

Take a look at monkeys, chimpanzees, and gorillas in the wild. These animals don't go to church, can't read the Bible, yet they live longer and healthier lives than we do. They don't carry around gym membership cards, nor are they members of Weight Watchers or Jenny Craig, yet they are healthier and live longer than we do. These wild animals don't have annual physicals, primary healthcare providers, or take prescription medications. Yet they can lift up to three times their own weight, and can reach 180 years in age without graying. It is interesting to note that their nutritional lifestyle mirrors the menu plan that was originally given to mankind in Genesis 1:29. These animals mostly eat seeded fruits, leaves, and herbs which are full of naturally alkalizing water, nutrients, essential fatty oils, vitamins, minerals, and a host of other healthy benefits. They maintain a constant balance of acidic and alkalizing foods in their diets.

If we want to save our faith, our wealth, our health, and our families, it would greatly benefit us if we were to implement some of the eating habits of these wild animals. As a matter of fact, today both the medical and scientific communities are saying the exact same thing. We are now told to eat at least four to five servings of fruits and vegetables every day and drink plenty of water. The Federal Government has just restructured the food pyramid which reflects the meal plan of the apes and chimpanzees.

Now it is time for all believers to wake up and be transformed by the renewing of your minds. Simply put, if it works for the animals, it will work for you. You are made in the image and likeness of God, not the animals. The animals' original role was the use of their blood to atone for the sins of mankind until Christ could once and for all accomplish this by dying on the cross. The following two scriptures point this out. Hebrews 9:22 says, "And almost all things are by the law purged with blood, and without shedding of blood is no remission." Hebrews 9:12 says, "Neither by the blood of goats and calves, but by his own blood he entered in once into the holy place, having obtained eternal redemption for us." Today, we simply consume too much meat which is highly contaminated with growth hormones, antibiotics, and poisonous chemicals added for commercial processing. Cooking meats at high temperatures produces even more toxic acids. Acid burns and destroys everything it comes in contact with, unless there is enough alkalinity to counter and stop it. The spiritual battle that is being waged against us is manifesting through the condition of our health, which greatly impacts our spiritual lives to include our faith.

Since man's creation, Satan has been at work to destroy him. Mankind's mission was to worship God and bring light into this present age of darkness, whose ruler is Satan. Matthew 5:14-16 says "You are the light of the world. Let your light shine before men, that they may see your good works and praise your father in heaven." After the fall of Satan and before the creation of the world, Ephesians 1:4, God decided to create an image of himself. This image of God mentioned in Genesis 1:16 "let us make man in our image," would be the light reflecting God's character, exposing the works of Satan in this present age of darkness. God knew that by putting man into this situation, it would be like sending soldiers off to war. So He created everything to support man first, and then topped it off with His magnanimous love and grace found in Ephesians. 1:6-11. However, God even went a step further and sealed man's redemption. 2nd Corinthians 5:18-21, just in case man was injured by sin, his injury wouldn't be hopeless or fatal. God put into place the sun, moon, and stars to support man.

He also placed life-sustaining minerals deep in the core of the earth to preserve man. Notice how God placed these resources far out of man's reach. Knowing that sin causes selfishness, He didn't want man to be able to control these life sustaining resources, and horde them for his own profit and gain. Just imagine we live in the 21st century, and man has yet to reach the sun or the core of the Earth. In fact, everything we know about these places are just an hypothesis, that's right, an educated guess. God was also well prepared and had a back-up plan for man's salvation and redemption. Plan A- the animals, who far outnumbered mankind at creation. The Bible teaches us that after Adam and Eve sinned, God forgave them and clothed them by sacrificing an animal, <u>Genesis 3:21, "God made garments of skin for Adam and his wife and clothed them."</u> Hebrews 9:22, <u>"Without the shedding of blood there is no forgiveness."</u> Plan B- Noah, a preacher of righteousness to unrepentant mankind 2nd Peter 2:5. Plan C- The Israelites taken out of the Gentile nations, <u>Psalms 80:8, "God brought a vine from out of Egypt."</u> Plan D- God himself, through the incarnation of his son Christ Jesus.

I want us to take a closer look at back-up Plan A- the animals. I want you to compare them to your child's college fund. We start saving for our children's college education when they are just innocent infants, and when the time comes to send them off to college, we tap into their college savings to help offset some of the cost. However, if instead of going to college, our child gets into trouble. This same college fund can now be used to save them by being diverted to pay for attorney and legal expenses.

So it was with the animals, God never intended for mankind to eat the animals according to <u>Genesis 1:29, "Then God said I give you every seed-bearing plant on the face of the whole earth, and every tree that has fruit with seed in it. They will be yours for food."</u> I want you to pay close attention to the words seed-bearing. These two words are of great significance in the intrinsic relationship between God and man. Man had no need for animals according to <u>Genesis 2:20, "but for Adam no suitable helper was found."</u> Genesis 3:7, <u>"Adam and Eve used fig leaves for clothing upon realizing they were naked."</u> So as you can plainly see, mankind did not depend on animal meat or protein for his survival. As a matter of fact, as part of man's pun-ishment, God added the plants originally given to the animals in Genesis 1:30 to man's diet, and not meat. So the animals were really here as a ransom whose blood would be used as a sacrificial atonement for mankind's sinful condition. This is where we derive the Old Testa-ment sacrificial practices first mentioned in Genesis, Chapter 4, and why Cain's sacrifices of fruit were not accepted by God. Because again, <u>Hebres 9:22, "without the shedding of blood there is no forgiveness."</u> Genesis 4:4, <u>"But Abel brought fat portions from some of the firstborn of his flock."</u> So the animals were the first ransom, and Christ was the final and ultimate ransom.

Now let's take a closer look at the seed-bearing fruits and trees mentioned in Genesis 1:29. If you were to cut open a piece of fruit, you will notice something very distinctive inside, the seed. The seed looks nothing like the fruit, yet the seed is really a separate living organism inside the fruit, with an inherent energy empowering it to produce the fruit we see. As the fruit develops, the seed inside is invisible to the naked eye. The seed will determine taste, color, smell, shape, and type of fruit. Fruit also contains the vitamins and minerals needed to preserve and sustain life, all of which come from the DNA of the seed. Seeds within the fruit produce phytonutrients which scientists are just now beginning to explore. Phytonutrients come from the Greek word phyton meaning a nutrient from a plant. The medical and scientific communities are finally confirming what our parents have always told us, "Eat your fruits and vegetables." The seeds of the fruit are power packed with nutrients that not only give fruits and vegetables their many colors, but also provide a lot of nature's natural medicines. The seed supplies the plants with the phytonutrients needed to preserve and promote optimum health.

There are three phytons that are commonly talked about: carotenoids, flavanoids, and isolavones. In actuality, there are probably thousands more that have not even been discovered yet. Scientists have just begun to tap into the medicinal powers of phytons over the past couple of years. These phytons are very effective in four distinct ways. To start with, they protect the body and fight disease. Have you ever watched a garden grow, and asked yourself how the plants stay so healthy. They are exposed to the elements, yet they don't wear sunscreens or raincoats. They don't have doctor visits or physical exams. The reason these plants remain healthy is due to the anti-disease fighting power produced from the seeds which nourish, protect, and preserve the plant. The same phytons that help keep the plant healthy also keep us healthy by providing medicine for the cells. These phytons help our cells repair themselves by releasing protective enzymes that rebuild damaged cells. They also inhibit cancer producing substances, reducing their ability to damage cells. Through prevention, degenerative diseases can stay in check and not overtake and debilitate the body.

Secondly, these phytonutrients are very effective in fighting cancer. We produce cancer cells almost everyday and normally the body fights them off. If the body's defenses are not strong enough due to over acidification, then we develop cancer. However, the protective properties from the seeds explain why Mediterranean cultures who consume tomatoes, cucumbers, garlic, fruits, onions, whole complete grains and olive oil, which are mostly alkalizing foods, have the lowest rates of cancer and heart disease. Numbers 11:4, speaks of the cucumbers, melons, leeks, onions, and garlic, again all alkalizing foods that the Israelites consumed in Egypt, which was balanced by the fish they consumed in abundance. Remember in an alkaline environment, disease and bacteria can't exist. These seed bearing plants also help the heart by keeping cholesterol levels in check.

Thirdly, the body's immune system is mobilized and starts to produce natural killer cells and helper-T cells. These act as protective armor helping to keep invading pollutants and bacteria from entering the cells. The fourth and most important role of these seed bearing fruits and plants is their ability to neutralize free radicals. Free radicals are vandal cells that attack and destroy normal cells. Seed bearing fruits and plants arrest the development and activity of free radicals. Satan understands the importance of seed bearing foods and how they can help to prevent, reverse, and even halt the progression of degenerative diseases. The seeds from pumpkins and grapefruit can kill parasites, worms, and control the growth of unhealthy bacteria. So he has corrupted the food supply in his attempt to counter God's instructions to us regarding our consumption of seed bearing herbs and fruits. Today, we have seedless fruits sold in our grocery stores and at produce stands. Genesis 1:29 says, "And God said, behold, I have given you every herb bearing seed, which is upon the face of all the earth, and every tree, in which is fruit of a tree yielding seed, to you it shall be for meat." Some of the most powerful disease fighting compounds on the face of the earth are contained in the seeds of certain fruits and herbs. The biggest problem with man-made medicine is we take the medications without it containing the seeds.

God's instructions in Gn.1:28 were to be fruitful first and then to multiply. God impregnated mankind with his spirit or seed, 1st Jn. 3:10, which would enable mankind to bare Godly fruitful character, this character being the visible expression of the invisible power producing it. In Gal.5:22, the first fruit of the Spirit is love. We know that love preserves and sustains life, fruit also preserves and sustains life. We cannot taste, see, or touch love because it is invisible. So God gave us fruit as a physical expression of His invisible character, Psalms 34:8, "Oh taste and see that the Lord is good. Blessed is the man who takes refuge in Him." So mankind's diet was a reflection of God's character. Now isn't it interesting to note that once man had fallen into sin, God, not man, decided to change the diet of mankind. Genesis 3:18 says, "Thorns also and thistles shall it bring forth for thee, and thou shall eat the herb of the field." No longer was man required to eat the seed-bearing herbs and fruit only. Man was now allowed to eat the food given to the animals mentioned in Gn.1:30. We know that sin separates us from God, so mankind no longer having God's seed in him would be able to bare Godly fruitful character. God would no longer invisibly empower man, so mankind no longer needed seed bearing herbs and fruit only as his diet. Plus, mankind didn't eat from the Tree of Life, so there was no need for him to continue eating just seed bearing herbs and fruits.

Mankind was given non-seed bearing herbs to supplement his vegetarian diet up until the time of Noah and the great flood. Here in Gn.9:3, God had flooded the earth, and Noah and his family had no vegetation to eat, so God allowed them to eat the clean animals which he instructed Noah to bring board the ark. Genesis 7:2 says, "Take with you seven pairs of every kind of clean animals and two of every kind of unclean animal." Now let us stop here for a second and digest clean and unclean. In Gn.7:1, it said that Noah was found righteous by God. In Lev.11:43, God instructs the Israelites not to allow themselves to become unclean by touching or eating any unclean animals. So Noah is instructed to bring more clean than unclean animals aboard the ark for two reasons: 1) He would need the clean animals to feed himself, his family, and make sacrifices. Genesis 8:20 says, "And Noah built an altar unto the Lord, and took of every clean beast, and of every clean fowl, and offered burnt offerings on the alter." The unclean animals would discard the dead carcasses of the clean animals to prevent the spread of disease and more importantly, so that Noah and his family would not defile themselves by eating or touching any unclean animals. 2) Because of man's sinful condition and his inability to produce Godly fruitful character, allowing mankind to live long in sin was undesirable to God. So man's years were shortened with the introduction of meat to his diet, with strict instructions not to eat the fat or blood, Lev.7:22.

So at creation, the Patriarchs lived well into the 900's, but nine generations after the creation of mankind, we're introduced to Methuselah, whose name means "when he dies the waters will come."

He dies at the age of 969, and then the earth was flooded. Noah survives the flood and lives to be 950, but just nine generations later, man is only reaching the age of 200, Gn.11:32. Man's longevity shortened precipitously after the addition of meat to his diet. Today, this would make a lot of sense being that meat causes the body to produce extra fat and cholesterol in the blood. Fat and cholesterol are connected to a myriad of degenerative diseases like cancer, diabetes, and heart disease. It also robs the body of energy during digestion, which leads to premature aging. The long list of ailments related to meat consumption reads like a medical text book. God gave permission to eat the clean animals only. The unclean animals were never to be eaten. These new dietary commandments given to Noah in Genesis, Chapter 9, were given hundreds of years before the Leviticul laws given to Moses at Mt. Sinai.

We must trust the Creator to know what is best for us to eat, instead of eating according to our own traditions. He not only made our bodies, but all the animals as well, and He certainly would not have made the distinction between "clean and unclean" if it didn't really matter what we ate. 1ˢᵗ Corinthians 10:31 sums it up beautifully, "Whether therefore ye eat, or drink, or whatever you do, do all to the glory of God and not to the glory of yourselves." I hear people saying to me all the time, "well, you know I have to die of something." I tell them that death has been a fact of life since the fall of Adam and Eve. Why not let God decide when that time will be for you instead of eating yourself into an early grave.

Remember, Satan wants to destroy the body, or temple where the Holy Spirit dwells. He desires for you to attach your faith to your health, which is temporal. Don't get me wrong, there is nothing wrong with wanting your body to be healed, but this body is just temporary, your faith is eternal. We are instructed to attach our faith to the ever-lasting and the non-temporal. Satan's ultimate mission is to prevent you from accomplishing the assignment that God has predestined for you, and to put out the light which exposes him for who he is in this present age of darkness.

The Lord desires order in the area of our physical condition. If it is not properly cared for, it affects our spiritual condition. We cannot serve the Lord to the fullest if our bodies are run down and tired, and not functioning as God designed them to function. The medical world is now recognizing that gluttony is one of the major causes of many of our modern day illnesses. Moderation should be your guide, Philippians 4:5, "Let your moderation be known unto all men. The Lord is at hand." You must fight back by making a conscious decision to eat healthier and exercise more. I pray that you will allow God to help you on this journey, so that you may live a happy, healthy, victorious life, and save yourself and your family. **Remember, God has placed before you life and death, sickness and disease, so choose life, that you and your seed may live.**

CHAPTER 8

The Physical Battles

"I have set before you life and death, blessing and cursing: therefore choose life, that both thou and thy seed may live:" (Deuteronomy 30:19)

Today, many of us follow traditions that have been in our families for generations. We practice the same generational habits and do things in pretty much the way our parents and grandparents did. We have recipes and use remedies that go back for decades, and believe it or not, some of these remedies are still very effective today. For instance when I was younger, my mom would always give us vinegar whenever we had heartburn. One day my mom had prepared collard greens for dinner. She cooked her greens southern style, using fat back and some old drippings that had been on top of the stove for a couple of weeks. I'll never forget that evening after eating the greens. At around two o'clock in the morning, I awoke with heartburn so severe, I actually thought I was going to die. The excruciating pain I was experiencing cramped my chest and stomach, so I couldn't stand straight or walk upright. I was only eight or nine at the time, and literally had to crawl from my bedroom and drag myself into the kitchen. I slowly and painfully pulled myself up to the pantry cabinet and got out the bottle of vinegar. Immediately, I swallowed two tea-spoons full, and within a few minutes, my condition had completely cleared up. All of the pain and agony I had been suffering just simply seemed to melt away. The vinegar was an old remedy passed down in my family for generations.

As much as I loved mom's cooking, I never ate her collard greens again. You see, she cooked with mineral-depleted table salt so my food lacked the proper balance of minerals needed to produce the stomach acids that would break down this meal for proper digestion and assimilation. Also, because the greens had been overcooked for hours, all of the healthy digestive enzymes were destroyed. As soon as the acid from the vinegar reached my stomach, it immediately started to settle things down and the pain subsided. I know my mom loved me and would never expose me to anything dangerous, but she was unknowingly causing my body more harm than good. Think about how many parents today feed their children every morning and happily send them off to school, unaware of the hidden health risk they are creating. Hundreds of millions of parents innocently poison their kids every day by feeding them pernicious foods they believe are actually healthy.

A typical morning breakfast starts out with a bowl of processed cereals containing up to 75% refined sugar, artificial chemical sweeteners, food colorings, and several other unreadable ingredients. It is fortified with cheap, synthetically-altered vitamins, minerals, and highly toxic refined table salt. We then add another health hazard known as pasturized milk to the most important meal of the day, which contains mutagenic substances, and is synthetically fortified with the same junk that's put into the cereal. This poisonous concoction is loaded with bioengineered hormones, gastrointestinal peptides, allergic proteins, antibiotics, bacteria, blood, pus, and growth inhibitors. It contains chemicals like Recombinant Bovine Growth Hormones (RBGH) made by Monsanto, the company who holds the patent on the now banned Agent Orange.

This milk-producing hormone causes udder infections in cows and has been banned in Europe and Canada. RBGH is especially harmful to children because it can cause constipation, chronic sniffles, colds, runny noses, and tonsillitis. This drug increases pus and bacteria counts in milk by 14%, and comes with a warning label that only dairy farmers get to read. In fact, dairy farmers won't even feed pasturized milk to their own baby calves because it will kill them. Now, because this synthetically man-made hormone causes dairy cows to overproduce an abundance of milk, generating more profits for the dairy industry at the risk of public health and safety, this poison is given to dairy cows and then passed on to us.

I know a young lady who, upon becoming a new mother, decided to breast-feed her little infant. Within a few weeks, she had to stop because the baby kept constantly throwing up her breast milk. She took her baby back and forth to the doctor for several tests to find out what was wrong. We prayed over the child on several occasions, but the problem continued to persist. It didn't take long though for doctors to determine that the baby could no longer drink the mother's milk and remain healthy. In fact, the breast milk was actually endangering the baby's life, because other illnesses were starting to adversely affect the child. This young lady would often consume as much as one gallon of milk per day. The infant could not handle the toxic side affects of the contaminants in the milk on her little body. Because she was only a few weeks old, her body was pretty much alkaline, which immediately rejected the breast milk. This alkaline condition enabled her immune system to properly protect her from the toxic chemicals passed to her from her mom. Many infants can no longer drink breast milk, with many having problems now consuming even baby formula. A lot of infants are overweight today because their bodies are toxic.

Two ways the body defends itself in regards to toxic poisoning is to retain excess water and produce excess fat. This is why a lot of woman have problems controlling their weight after going on birth control medications. These drugs toxify the body so it uses both defenses to protect itself from the toxic affects of birth control pills. Women who stop taking birth control usually notice an immediate drop in their weight. God created an all-natural birth control solution for married couples that causes no toxic side affects. God has designed it so that a woman is only fertile between two to six days in the month. Known as the rhythm method, it has worked very effectively in my marriage for the past 15 years.

As if enough damage hasn't been done already to start out the morning, we top this off by giving them a tall glass of fruit juice, juice that has been completely stripped of all its naturally occurring minerals, vitamins, and fiber which is vitally important to human health. When fiber is present in our foods, blood sugars rise at a much slower and safer rate. Fiber is also very effective in keeping the digestive system clean, by gently sweeping and collecting excess waste for removal from the body. This is, sadly, how the average American child starts out their day, and are expected to function in their right mind. Without consuming the natural minerals, vitamins and other nutrients that God commanded mankind to eat, it is amazing that they can function at all. How can these poor little innocent children remain healthy without eating the health preserving phytonutrients that God placed into seed bearing fruits and herbs. This easily explains why America consumes more food and uses more prescriptive medications than any other country on the face of the earth. Yet government studies have shown that up to 95% of this country's population is suffering from malnutrition.

Don't blame your children for the way they behave; put the blame on yourself. You may think that you are innocent, but that doesn't change the status of your child's health. If you don't pay your utility bills, you'll quickly be in the dark. If you remove the detergent from the laundry cleanser, all you have is a solution of dyes and perfumes. No matter how great it smells, it will not clean your clothes. If you don't sow into your body what it needs to properly function, it will be in the dark also.

As I said earlier, I come from a very large family of twenty four aunts and uncles, and that's just on my mom's side. My grandparents were very poor, and couldn't afford to go to the doctor every time one of their children became ill. So they had to use whatever they could get their hands on, and if it worked, it stayed around. I remember a few years back attending one of my son's basketball games at the local YMCA. Upon entering the gymnasium, I noticed a woman sitting in the bleachers with a large white towel in her hands. Her eyes were blood shot red, teary, and swollen. She continuously wiped her irritated, dripping nose as she sat looking totally miserable. I hesitated for a moment before sitting down, because I had my little three-year-old daughter with me, and I didn't know how safe it would be. Since the gym was very crowded, I decided to take a seat next to hers.

As we began to talk, she started explaining to me that she had suffered for many years with severe allergies. Her sinuses dripped all the time, so she carried the towel around because none of the medications she took relieved her condition. I asked what type of foods she ate on a regular basis, and was she eating eggs or dairy. She told me that she ate as many as four to six eggs everyday and used quite a bit of mayonnaise. I suggested that she stop eating the eggs and any products containing eggs or dairy. I gave her a daily detox to drink that included raw lemon, distilled water, cayenne pepper, and pure maple syrup. I told her to drink this twice daily until her symptoms totally cleared up. The following week when I walked into the gym, I could not believe my eyes. I could hardly recognize this woman from just one week earlier. The hand towel was gone and her nose and eyes looked totally normal. I could see a spark of excitement in her eyes as if she had just found a new lease on life.

She must have thanked God for sending me her way for about a half an hour. She was in total shock, and couldn't believe that all these years she had lived in bondage and thought there was no hope. She told me that her mother and grandmother also suffered with sinus problems for decades. It completely baffled her that something so simple and cheap as lemon and water could reverse a decades old condition that had been passed down in her family for generations. When I saw her a year later, she was still sinus free and reminded me about that faithful day we met in the gym. Why did the detox work? Because God had ordained it to work before he created the foundation of the earth. Lemons contain 27 natural anti-bacterial compounds that attack and kill bacteria, and is also one of the top alkalizers, with water and maple syrup following next in line.

Her sinus problem was a direct result of her acidic generational dietary habits. The continuous nose drainage was her body's way of throwing out the toxins produced from this acidic condition. Once she alkalized her blood and removed the highly acidic foods from her diet, her body immediately responded, even after decades of being out of balance. My point is simply this, only God has the final say regarding your health, not medical science or any human being. When man says no, God says yes. The wonderful thing about God is the fact that what He has created does not need any type of human testing. Everything He created was brought into existence by His word. He says that heaven and earth shall pass away, but His word will stand forever.

Today, many people have allergic reactions to certain types of seeded fruits and herbs. This is because they are already overly acidic to begin with. These acidic conditions can be passed on from parents to their infants, depending on the condition of the previous parents blood. I once witnessed this happen to my nephew, who was born with the same type of acidic skin condition as his parents. The good thing is that all hereditary degenerative diseases are reversible, but first the body has to be brought into the right internal state to heal itself. By the way, if you are allergic to shellfish, that's a good thing, because you shouldn't be eating those types of foods to begin with. They were never meant for human consumption, and are highly toxic and rich in artery clogging cholesterol.

I have seen many instances where people have recovered totally from inherited diseases once they took their health seriously. Today, we use antacids like Tums and Rolaids to treat indigestion which, in the grand scheme of things, really makes no sense. Our bodies naturally create digestive acids when we eat to help break down our food before it can be absorbed through the intestines. Whatever you eat, fried chicken, steak, ice cream, cookies, crackers, fruits, vegetables, etc., it all has to be broken down and absorbed through the intestines before the body can benefit from it. The production of these acids to help aid digestion are so imperative to the overall state of your health. This is why taking antacids, which blocks acid production in the stomach, is so dangerously unhealthy. Without these acids, our food simply spoils in our intestines and begins to rot and putrefy.

To make matters worse, just about everyone drinks some type of sugary liquid, like soda, cool aid, or fruit punch with their meals. This greatly complicates matters because these drinks are highly acidic and oxygen depleting, they contain no fiber, and insidiously leach the bones of precious minerals. As your food rots in your gut, it begins to ferment in this sugary, highly acidic, oxygen lacking, mold infested, bacteria producing, parasitic thriving environment. The dinner you just ate now becomes dinner for the billions of other unhealthy bacteria who are always fighting to take control of your health. They must eat also, and as your body is starved to death of the oxygen, vitamins, minerals, and nutrients it needs for optimal health, these uninvited guests leave behind toxic waste material that poisons the blood. This brings about internal system breakdown followed by multiple organ malfunctions.

The simple absence of digestive acids starts a crippling chain of events which now affect the body's ability to defend itself. No matter how much food you eat, without stomach acids, properly balanced minerals, and living enzymes, it is absolutely impossible for digestion to take place. Your tiny microscopic cells can't absorb a hamburger and fries, in the same way you cannot eat a whole cow unless it is first butchered. The immune and endocrine systems are both compromised and disabled because the organs that support them are diseased due to degenerating conditions of the cells that support these organs. This allows unhealthy bacteria to take hold of the body and deteriorate your health. It is where the fight for life and death starts and ends. If this condition is not corrected over time, systems failure spreads throughout the entire body causing sickness, disease, and eventually premature death. I can't stress enough the importance of proper nutrition, digestion, and assimilation. Some things are just worth repeating. Unless you have unrefined, mineral-rich sea salt with all your meals, digestion is all but impossible. In the same way your body parts interact with each other, minerals are dependent upon each other for optimum performance.

A lot of times, indigestion problems can be alleviated by simply eating properly salted foods in their right combinations. We simply eat too many of the wrong types of mineral-depleting foods together, and then wash them down with a poisonous sugary drink. How can you drink poison and expect not to suffer any adverse reactions. I remember once climbing up unto the kitchen counter, and there I discovered a cup of clear liquid of what I thought to be soda. Without hesitating, I drank from the cup and immediately started gagging and throwing up. What I thought was one thing was actually a cup of poisonous Clorox bleach. Now my reaction to the bleach was immediate, unlike refined sugar which is just as deadly, but works slower and more insidiously as it defiles your blood and destroys your organs. You see, sugar causes catastrophic damage over a longer period of time. Sugar is not a real food and contains empty calories. So the body is tricked into believing it is actually being fed, when in reality it isn't. Once the brain realizes it has been hoodwinked and bamboozled, it orders the body to seek out real nutrients. Overeating is the result of our body's craving for real food to supply its energy needs. If you were eating whole foods that were properly digested and producing the proper sugars needed by the body, you wouldn't overeat.

This is also where exercise plays a major role because of the hormone dopamine. Have you ever been hungry but instead of eating, you worked out. You probably noticed that your desire to eat suddenly disappeared. This happens because exercising forces a large amount of this hormone to be released into the blood. Dopamine, a chemical naturally produced in the body, gives the brain a feeling of satisfaction and pleasure. With this hormone present, the brain no longer senses the need to eat so food cravings stop. Water content is also very important. If your food is more water soluble, it will contain more oxygen, and you wouldn't feel as if you were choking while you eat. The desire to drink liquids with your meals would no longer be a matter of life and death. Plus water would stop the destruction of vital nutrients by preventing over acidification in the stomach. What is more amazing is the fact that eating foods in their proper combinations and types is the most effective way to lose weight and keep it off permanently. If you are struggling with weight issues, drink a glass of water before you eat and sip on water as you eat.

You may think that the food you're eating today is the same quality that your parents and grandparents had. There is a huge difference. The foods of their day were real, while the foods we eat today are synthetically engineered. Their food was much fresher than ours, and the soil the food grew in was much more mineral rich. The farming soils of this country have been totally defiled and corrupted by the heavy use of artificial fertilizers which over acidify the ground. Originally, our bodies received the minerals it needed from two sources- plants and salt. The plants received their minerals from the soil. We then ate the plants, as grains, vegetables and fruits. Just in the last 50 years, mankind has introduced artificial fertilizers. This has allowed the cultivation of larger areas of land increasing in yield per acre, and greatly improved productivity. However, the artificial fertilizer does not replace the 80 or so minerals the plants took in from the soil. So our soils have become mineral depleted. Studies show that the vegetables of today contain only 10% of the nutrition of vegetables grown just 50 years ago. Between 1950 and 1975, the calcium content in one cup of rice dropped 21%, iron fell by 28.6%, and protein content dropped nearly 11%. In 1945, wheat was 17% protein, but by 1985, its protein content dropped to 9%.

Now it is very important that you clearly understand what type of warfare is taking place here. With the plague of people suffering with degenerative diseases in this country, one would think this was a third-world nation. Sadly, every 30 seconds someone dies from heart disease, every 55 seconds another dies of cancer, every third person has an allergic reaction to something, every 13 minutes a woman dies from breast cancer, and every fifth person is mentally ill. The brain requires a vast array of nutrients, vitamins, minerals and amino acids to produce the chemicals needed for proper cell to cell communication. Just the absence of one mineral can greatly alter this function which can result in diminished mental capacity and emotional instability. This includes behavioral disorders such as depression, autism, anxiety, hyperactivity, eating disorders, drug and alcohol addiction, attention deficit disorder, and violence to name a few.

In the early 1980s, a research report was reprinted entitled "The Impact of a Low Food Additive and Sucrose Diet on Academic Performance in 803 New York City Schools." From 1980 to 1983, major dietary policy revisions were made with regard to the use of sucrose, fats and food additives. During the four-year period in which these food factors were reduced in the diet of the school children, the mean national academic performance of the 803 schools rose from 41% to 51%. This resulted in NYC schools moving from 11% below the national average to 5% above it. A "reduction in malnutrition" was cited by the researchers as the cause of the rise. Everyone in this country is suffering from malnutrition because of our mineral depleted soils. The spiritual battle for your existence is taking place with every meal you eat.

Here is a true lesson in Tactical Warfare 101. The success of any war is not determined by the size or strength of the opposing forces, but by the successful art of deception. Go back and study every triumphant military campaign in the history of mankind, and you will find this to be the case. The great city of Troy, whose walls could not be penetrated by much larger and more powerful armies, were breached through the mastery of deception. Hitler tricked Russia and Germany's other neighboring allies during WWII. In the end, Hitler was deceived by the weather, and the most powerful army in the world at the time was defeated. The United States military, being out-numbered 4 to1, was able to annihilate thousands of well fortified and entrenched Japanese soldiers through the art of deception. The recent war against Iraq opened with an ambiguous beach assault that totally threw the enemy off guard. Yes, whoever masters the art of deception will always win the battle as it relates to human terms. Remember, God cannot be deceived. Deception requires very careful planning and thorough preparation. If you know the modes of operation of your enemy, his weaknesses and strengths, through ambiguity one can easily counter his advances.

Now Satan is our adversary, and he realizes that some of us love food more than we love God. He was created full of wisdom and perfect in beauty. Having years of experience on his resume, we are totally out matched by him in regards to the art of warfare without having God in our lives. The purpose of deception is to use trickery to conceal the real strategy or intentions of the adversary. If he can get all of your attention focused in one area, then he can attack through other exposed flanks. He will never have to change his strategy until you figure out his tactics. This is where the art of spiritual warfare gets very complicated for those who are always looking in one direction. Many people want to blame the problems in our society on unseen spiritual forces, while totally ignoring very real physical issues.

As long as Satan can get us to devote all of our energy in one direction, he can continue to attack and cripple society. Satan knows that each of us, upon death, must spiritually return back to God, and cannot freely roam about in the earth. As long as your soul doesn't have a body to operate in, there isn't anything you can do to disrupt his evil works. So his plan is to attack your physical body through disability or by premature death. In essence, while the church is focusing its energies on combating unseen spiritual forces, it is physically being destroyed by a myriad of visible preventable degenerative diseases.

For example, in 2002, 1.2 million men died in this country, 80% of them died of heart disease. Today, cancer is the leading cause of death for all Americans under the age of 85. That's roughly 98.6% of the total population. One-third of all cancer deaths are a direct result of smoking, which again is highly preventable. One out of every two women will die of heart disease. Here's another way of putting this. For every two women reading this book, one will die of heart disease. Nearly 62 million Americans have diabetes or pre-diabetes, and almost half don't even know it. One million new cases of diabetes are diagnosed every year, with a half of million people dying annually. This year, almost one million people will suffer a new or recurrent stroke, with African American women rising steadily in the ranks. An estimated 127 million Americans are overweight or obese. This statement can be easily validated by simply attending a regular Sunday service or social gathering. I want to remind you again that over two-thirds of these deaths and degenerative diseases are totally preventable. According to doctors at both the AHA and the ACS, an additional 250,000 people die annually due to iatrogenic (medical malpractice) causes in this country.

All of the statistics given above include just as many believers as non-believers. Degenerative diseases have no respect of person; they rain on the just as well as the unjust. This year alone, I personally know of four pastors who lost their wives to cancer and heart disease. Satan fully understands the fact that just because you don't profess Christ today, it doesn't mean you will not profess him in the future.

Case in point was the Apostle Paul before being converted. The strategy is to destroy those who are currently serving God, and also those who may come into the faith later in life. I've only listed here the five major causes of death which, by the way, are all preventable. Satan knows they are preventable, and he understands that as long as he can keep you thinking that they're not, your attention will remain diverted and focused on other counterfeit tactics. He wants you to believe that the counterfeit is bigger than what it actually is, in the same way he wants you to believe that he is bigger and more powerful than God. Through these cunning devices, he has mastered the art of deceptive warfare over our lives. The church has focused the majority of its efforts to combat dark unseen spiritual forces in heavenly places while its members standby and helplessly watch themselves and their loved ones needlessly suffer, and die prematurely here on the earth.

The book of Daniel speaks of a battle that was fought in the heavenly realm by opposing unseen spiritual forces. The outcome of all earthly battles are determined by the successes or failures of opposing angelic forces in heavenly places. In Daniel's case, the angel was detained 21 days by the Prince of Persia before receiving aid from the archangel Gabriel. Thus the battles in heavenly places can be won or lost. During these 21 days of battle, Daniel did not participate in the struggle against the Prince of Persia. He was physically ill himself. We ought to take our cue from Daniel and leave the spiritual warfare to the heavenly forces who are equipped to deal with them while we simply put on the whole armor of God and stand, following the lead of the Holy Spirit who will teach and guide us regarding all matters, enabling us to save ourselves, family, and friends so we can further the work of Christ here on the earth.

Being a musician, I often get to meet and accompany very interesting and powerful individuals. I remember playing for this powerful woman of God who came to speak for a special service. She had everyone clapping, standing to their feet, and just all riled up. People were falling out all over the place as she laid hands and gave a prophetic word. After the service, my wife and I gave her a ride home since her car was in the repair shop. Before we could get into my car, she started complaining about her sinuses, aching joints, migraine headaches, and other physical ailments. She asked me if I wouldn't mind stopping at the drugstore so that she could get her pain medicine and other medications. She must have been taking five or six different medications for a whole list of ailments. I thought to myself, my God! How can you have a word for everybody else and not one for yourself. The offering she received for speaking was now leaving the body of Christ. She was slightly on the heavy side, and admitted that her passion for food was getting the best of her. In other words, food had become her God, and she was suffering miserably because of it. 1ˢᵗ Corinthians 3:16-17 says, "Do you not know that you are the temple of God and that the spirit of God dwells in you. If anyone defiles the temple of God, God will destroy him. For the temple of God is Holy, which temple are you."

As I visit churches around this country, I realized this poor woman is not alone. I once spoke at a church and just about 90% of the congregation had some type of affliction, or were taking prescription drugs. As I listened to one person after another, I heard the same hopelessness and dread in each of their voices. What really stuck in my mind most was the disproportionate number of young people, just reaching into their teens, who were suffering with degenerative diseases and taking medications. Why isn't the Holy Spirit sending a word to save our innocent children who are not just sick, but are dying in record numbers. They were born having to fight for their lives, before ever taking their first steps. There are so many prosperity messages and prophecies going around today. Now true prosperity is not how much money God is going to send you, because no amount of money can buy you health. What's the use of having a lot of prosperity and wealth if you have to spend it all on healthcare. What's the use of having prosperity if your children are sick and debilitated. The key is to have health and wealth together. Fight against the war that is prematurely crippling and taking the lives of so many believers everyday, destroying their health and stealing their wealth.

When I became an investment banker, I sat through a pep speech one morning about how important it was to make as much money as possible. We were told how money can buy you the best things in life, including the best medical care. How money can supply all of your needs. As long as you have money, you can control and empower your destiny. The entire room was pumped and excited about the prospect of being empowered through wealth. The speaker was very wealthy himself, and spoke about how he had an infant child who was gravely ill. He suggested that his riches afforded him access to the best medical practitioners in the world. He stated that there was absolutely nothing he wouldn't give or do for his child. Yet in the end, all the money and medical experts on the planet could not save his child's life. Prosperity without the health to enjoy it is like having no prosperity at all.

Land ownership is very important to God and Satan knows this. You are a very valuable piece of mobile real estate. God has declared that the earth is His and the fullness thereof. Every time you move about the earth in right relationship with God, you validate His word. Look at every commandment concerning land that God gave to Adam, Noah, Abraham, the Israelites, and even Jesus telling His disciples to go out into all the earth. When you and God are walking together, you are instantly worth more than all of the combined real estate in Beverly Hills because you have the ability to change and positively impact the lives of others. The last thing Satan wants to acknowledge is that God owns anything that can slow his progression of evilness. So through greed he has defiled the soil, which has corrupted our food supply. What was once a highly valuable piece of real estate declines in value into a diseased and dysfunctional plot of land. Colossians 4:6 says, "Let your speech always be with grace, seasoned with salt, that you may know how to answer each other." The salt mentioned here is not mineral-depleted table salt, but real mineralized salt that God has balanced through nature.

By removing minerals from the salt and soil, Satan has destroyed the only two sources of naturally occurring minerals for all humans, animals, and plants. Everyone is affected and each succeeding generation is adversely impacted, resulting in increased incidents of degenerative diseases and mental disorders. Today, people will take you out just for simply looking at them the so-called "wrong" way. You can easily lose your life by simply crossing into someone else's lane of traffic without signaling. Everyone is on edge and so easily provoked at the slightest incitement.

Everyone is lacking vital minerals necessary for brain function like lithium, chromium and vanadium, and are prone to develop powerful salt or sugar cravings. Refined sugar and table salt leaches minerals from the blood and reserves in the marrow of the bones, therefore deepening the deficiency. Vitamins, proteins, enzymes, amino acids, as well as fats and carbohydrates, require minerals to work in the body making minerals the most needed nutrient of all. Fertilizers acidify the soil destroying microorganisms whose job it is to transform soil minerals into a form that is usable by plants. In the absence of this process, plants absorb dangerous amounts of heavy metals that are then passed on to us. These plants are also deficient in vitamins and proteins, which are required to make the neurotransmitters necessary for cells to communicate.

Today, many children are being born diseased and mineral deficient, because their parents are passing along to them genes that are defective and sick. Look at the undeniable difference between infants who are raised on breast milk and those fed baby formula. Non-breast fed babies suffer with more virile infections, adolescent weight problems, and have a lower I.Q. than those raised on breast milk. This alone proves that if certain elements are missing from what God has ordained to keep us healthy, physical and mental disabilities will manifest. A mother's breast milk was designed by God, not by some scientist sitting in a laboratory. No human mind can outmatch the mind of God when it comes to creating something perfect. Expectant moms here in America receive some of the best so-called prenatal care available. Yet the breast milk of tribal African mothers is healthier than the breast milk fed to infants in this country. American moms are mineral deficient and it reflects in their breast milk even though they take prenatal vitamins and minerals during their pregnancies. The tribal moms living in the jungles of Africa never take prenatal supplements nor do they have monthly checkups.

Fruits and vegetables are harvested before they have fully developed, when their mineral and vitamin content is low. Just about everything we eat has been bleached, colored, enriched, preserved, or refined. Only a minimal amount of our food is natural, fresh, or raw. We are now pumping our bodies full of poisonous sugars, artificial sweeteners, and heavy toxic metals, not taking in any of the naturally balanced minerals that God created to make us function. We don't really have to look very far to see why so many people are suffering from a myriad of illnesses. What is more frightening is that today, many people are dying from multiple illnesses simultaneously. We are so extremely spiritual-minded, yet we neglect our bodies by overeating and lack of exercise. We have been tricked into believing that because we were born with an inherited ailment, we have to suffer and live with it when we're actually supposed to be new creatures with a transformed mind.

When I was in elementary school, my mother was once told by our family physician that all nine of her children would have to take high blood pressure medication the rest of our lives, because we inherited hypertension from my father. Out of all nine siblings, I was the only one who never took any medication or suffered with high blood pressure. How is this possible? How was I able to dodge this degenerative generational bullet? What made me so different from everyone else? I am convinced that the Holy Spirit was leading me early in life to change unhealthy generational habits, knowing one day I would need to give this testimony. Also making healthier dietary choices and exercising early in my life has had a huge positive impact.

The enemy has us preaching to others about not fornicating, committing adultery, lying, and stealing. We are constantly judging and watching what others do. Now who is watching us and the sins we commit with the fork, spoon, and our bad eating habits? Can't you see it's all just a diversion? Many of us can no longer eat the original diet that God gave us of fruits and vegetables because of allergic reactions. Yet we can fill our stomachs with all kinds of toxic unclean foods, highly acidic sugary soft drinks, and then simply pop a pill. The only problem is that most medications have toxic side affects themselves that are damaging to both the liver and kidneys, the vital organs that cleanse our three internal oceans of body fluids. Look how well the enemy is deceiving us, yes us believers too. While we are looking to the right, Satan is blind siding us from the left with deadly delectable temptations. He shows us the fried chicken, but not the cancerous fat molecules, brain poisoning aluminum, and indigestible toxic proteins. You see the chocolate cake, but not the deadly saturated fat, or the artery clogging cholesterol.

It is imperative that foods be eaten in their proper combinations to be properly digested and assimilated into the body. For example, it takes two different types of enzymes to break down proteins and starches. When these enzymes come into contact with each other in the stomach, they cancel each other out. Therefore, the food in your stomach is not processed. Your entire meal basically spoils and is forced into your intestines. There it ferments and turns into a breeding ground for all kinds of bacteria and parasites. These parasites will attach themselves to your intestinal walls, and start the slow destruction of your health. You will be forced to overeat and crave minerals because your body is trying to survive.

The process of cell regeneration is perpetual. Every day, your body sheds billions of cells and grows billions back. Your body needs minerals in order to produce these cells. We absorb minerals after our food is properly digested through proper enzyme activity. The natural enzymes in our food and bodies work together so the body can save energy during digestion. This will, in turn, slow down the aging process, and you won't feel sluggish and sleepy after each meal. All digestion breaks down food into basic sugars or at least it should. If your food is improperly digested, your digestion process does not manifest these sugars and you develop sugar cravings.

Listen, I don't expect you to change your eating habits, because of what I say. 1st Thessalonians 5:21 says, "To prove all things and hold fast to that which is good." This life change is a gradual process, but I do encourage you to let moderation be your guide. You didn't wake up suddenly sixty pounds overweight. All of the minerals stored in your bones were not depleted in one day. No one develops heart disease over night. This process takes years to manifest. It took time for your body to get out of shape, and it will take time to get it back into shape. So don't be too anxious. Try to change a little bit everyday, and before you know it, you will be healthier and happier than you've ever been, and so will your children and your loved ones.

As your body replenishes its mineral reservoirs, amazing things will start to happen. You will no longer crave sugar or overeat. You will feel more relaxed and have more energy. It took many years for me to learn how to properly nourish and care for this temple. I first had to stop believing all the lies that we're bombarded with by the food advertisers and do some thorough investigating myself. Most importantly, I had to listen when my body was trying to tell me that things weren't okay. Your body will try to give you early warning signals. It's up to you to pay attention and make the needed changes. I once ate a piece of ham when I was younger. As soon as I ate the ham, my head started throbbing as if I was being hit with a hammer. I became dizzy and almost passed out. It even frightened my mom.

She immediately knew my blood pressure had gone up, and told me I couldn't eat pork anymore. My body was letting me know it couldn't handle the pork so I listened. I haven't eaten a piece since.

In cars where the engine oil is changed regularly, the engine will last for hundreds of thousands of miles. However, if the same engine never receives clean oil, it may last fifteen to twenty thousand miles before he engine locks up and the car dies. As new as the car is, with a dead engine, the car is not going very far. Your body is no different. Without consuming live nutrients and drinking clean water, your body's internal engines die. We are prepared and have resigned ourselves to expect our young people to suffer with frequent headaches, digestive disorders, nervous tension, insomnia, decaying teeth, and respiratory ailments. We expect them to be overweight by the time they reach grade school, and incapable of running a few yards or walking a few miles without suffering from exhaustion.

During one Christmas holiday, I went out shopping and took my own survey. I found that for every normal weight person I saw, there were three to four persons overweight. You may ask yourselves why I talk about being overweight so much. The answer is very simple. This problem is inextricably connected to five major degenerative diseases. A very large percentage of people develop heart disease, cancer, hypertension, diabetes, and obesity as they gain weight. With that said, some people instead of gaining visible weight, grow fat around their internal organs, which is just as deadly.

Losing weight through the use of diet pills does not make you a healthier person overall. You must control weight issues through proper exercise and consistent internal cleansing. Unseen fat surrounding the heart will eventually lead to heart disease and premature death. People are willing to take drastic measures like gastric by-pass surgery to remove unwanted body fat. This operation is very dangerous, with up to 50% of those undergoing such procedures dying within the first couple of years. You must control your weight through healthy lifestyle choices, not by taking short cuts. In the end, you will pay in one way or another. I want you to understand the fact that losing weight is not healthy if it doesn't heal the body also **Remember, God has placed before you life and death, sickness and disease, so choose life, that you and your seed may live**.

C H A P T E R   9

The Healthy Woman

"I have set before you life and death, blessing and cursing: therefore choose life, that both thou and thy seed may live" (Deuteronomy 30:19)

Genesis 2:22 says, "And the rib which the Lord God had taken from the man, made He a woman, and brought her unto the man." We later learned that she would be responsible for birthing new life into the earth. This process hasn't changed since that fateful day. Women remain vitally important to the existence of mankind. It would be fitting that if women were no longer able to procreate, humanity as we know it would vanish. With this prospect in mind, I decided to devote a chapter to the most important species on the face of the entire earth. Could you imagine living in a world without her gentle, soothing, colorful, encouraging, thoughtful, long suffering and nourishing character. What a desolate and empty place this world would become without her loving and nourishing nature. If you were to ask a group of women what they fear most in life as it relates to their health, the majority of them would say dying from breast cancer or AIDS. Heart disease and stroke would probably be last on their list of greatest concerns. According to statistics and research compiled over the past 21 years, the number one cause of death for women, especially above the age of 25, is heart disease, with strokes running close behind.

Researchers at Harvard Medical School and the American Heart Association say that heart disease claims twice as many women's lives as all forms of cancer combined. In fact, breast cancer claims 40,000 women annually, which doesn't even come close to the 499,000 women who die of heart disease every year. That's more than ten times the amount caused by breast cancer. What is more alarming is that these numbers are not falling, but steadily rising. I don't want to devote this entire chapter to just heart disease. How ever since it is the number one killer of women and kills women in such large numbers, I felt compelled to help raise the awareness about this silent but deadly killer. Far too many women think that heart disease is just a man's disease. Conventional wisdom says that more men suffer from heart disease than women; however, just the opposite is true. In fact, every year since 1984, more women have died from heart disease than men. Of all the preventable degenerative diseases that exist, heart disease is by far the easiest to prevent. With proper nutrition, exercise, and lifestyle choices, women can help protect themselves against heart disease.

This chapter will help women arm themselves with the information and knowledge they will need to reverse and prevent this silent killer. The reason it's considered a silent killer is because more that 65% of all women who suffer heart attacks never have any advance warnings or symptoms. There are roughly 10 million women who currently have heart disease, and probably another 10 to 15 million who are starting to develop the condition. Most women think their biggest threat is breast cancer or AIDS. These threats are small in comparison to their bigger enemies. A majority of women's death certificates list two diseases that are normally only associated with men. They report that two out of every five women actually die from heart disease and stroke. In fact, every minute in this country a woman dies from heart disease. What is really disheartening is the fact that these women are getting younger and younger. As I stated earlier, women as young as 25 years of age are having heart attacks in record numbers according to researchers at the Harvard Medical School.

Considering the fact that women haven't changed in their physical make up since being taken out of the man, paintings discovered by archeologist on the walls of pre-historic caves dating back several thousands years depict women giving birth pretty much the same way they do today, of course without all of the lights and glitter. Now my point is this, if the physical anatomy of a woman's body hasn't changed in the past 6000 years, then what has? The food that we consume on a daily basis is not what our ancestors ate in any way, shape, or form. In addition to the food is the lack of physical activity which again, I cannot stress the importance of. If you expect to live healthy for any length of time, you had better get active as soon as possible. In past times, recommending exercise for patients diagnosed with heart disease or who had suffered a heart attack was considered taboo. That type of thought is now considered a myth. If you have been diagnosed with heart disease, it is more important than ever to exercise. No longer is bed rest for weeks at a time the norm for heart attack victims. They are now encouraged to start exercising and moving about as soon as possible, even before being discharged from the hospital. The human body needs to exercise in order for the heart, arteries, and veins to remain healthy. It doesn't matter if you walk briskly for just 30 minutes four to five times a week. The walking will force your larger muscle groups to squeeze and contract your lymph glands. This squeezing and contracting motion will force these glands to cleanse and recycle your blood, removing a lot of the garbage that leads to heart disease in the first place.

Is exercise the only factor? Of course not. I'll get to what I believe is the biggest culprit in a minute. First, I want to dispel a few more myths that are causing this condition to go unchecked and hampering ways to effectively deal with this epidemic. With this disease taking the lives of almost 500,000 women annually, it's definitely time to pay attention and start making some lifestyle changes for the entire family. Most of the attention over the past years has primarily focused on men when it comes to heart disease. With the majority of the population thinking that breast cancer was the greatest threat facing women, I must admit that even I was taken by surprise when I learned that this was not the case. Again, I'll repeat statistics. One out of every two women die of heart disease. For every minute that passes, we lose another mother, sister, aunt, niece, or grandmother.

I hope you see why this issue must be immediately addressed. We don't have any extra minutes to spare. With 38% of women dying within their first year of having a heart attack, and 35% suffering a second heart attack within the same year, time is truly of the essence. Even with intervention, women are twice as likely to die from by-pass surgery than men. According to researchers, women's heart attacks seem to be far more fatal than men's. It is hard to believe that those responsible for bringing life into the world are being attacked and taken out the world before their children can reach grade school. For those women who do make it to experience menopause, their heart disease risks start to rise significantly. Many women have a difficult time interpreting the early signs of heart trouble because they can mimic other conditions like indigestion, acid reflux, anxiety, depression, shortness of breath, and fatigue. There is some good news that comes out of all of this. This disease is directly connected to unhealthy lifestyle choices, which can easily be altered to stop and reverse this deadly epidemic. I lost my mom to brain cancer at the age of 19. While I thank God for the 19 wonderful years I had to spend with her, I still miss her a great deal. Young people, you should love and cherish every precious moment you have with your moms. I know you may not agree with her all the time, but believe me, she deserves all the respect and love you can give her. What I wouldn't give to have my mother around today to see her grand-children or just to hear her comforting voice. Hey, I'm sorry, but you never truly realize how much they mean to you until they are gone.

Okay, now we can get down to the business of reversing this disease. As I stated earlier, I believe that through the art of deception, we have been tricked again. We have been told that salt is unhealthy and fat is bad for us. However, we've not been informed that there are certain good fats like essential fatty acids (EFAs) and minerals in real unrefined Celtic Sea Salt that our bodies cannot function without. These two foods regulate three of the most vital areas within the body: the heart, brain and immune system. Your body is totally useless without the proper function of these necessary components.

We've been looking at salt for too long as something to season our foods with instead of a substance to resupply our bodies with vitally important minerals. Our life sustaining substances, EFAs, in the form of Omega 3-6-9 oils, and mineral rich salts have been stripped of their nutritional benefits, and transformed into deadly counterfeits. All for the love of money. Our food industry has been used by Satan to cause a famine in our bodies. That's right. Americans may look healthy and wealthy, but we're the sickest people on the planet. So the body of Christ has been deceived while following the rest of the world and is suffering the same afflictions. The three deadly counterfeits are refined sugar, mineral-depleted table salt, and hydrogenated oils (non-EFA).

This deadly cocktail destroys both the physical and mental capacity of mankind. Not only is the sugar dangerous and the salt deadly, but we're also consuming too many unhealthy fats. Yes, believe it or not there are "good" and "bad" fats. Bad fats are the saturated fats found in red meat, butter, cream, milk, and cheese, and trans fats found in margarine. Saturated fats and trans fats can be converted to body fat, can harden the arteries, raise blood pressure, and contribute to cancer and diabetes. Good fats, on the other hand, are found in flaxseed oil, flax seeds, flaxseed meal, olive oil, olives, borage oil, evening primrose oil, black currant seed oil, hemp seed oil, hemp seeds, walnuts, pumpkin seeds, Brazil nuts, sesame seeds, avocados, some dark leafy green vegetables (kale, spinach, purslane, mustard greens, collards, etc.), canola oil (cold-pressed and unrefined), soybean oil, wheat germ oil, salmon, mackerel, sardines, anchovies, chestnut oil, and chicken. Without EFAs, the "good" fats in your diet, you could not think, see, hear, reproduce, run or even move a muscle. Hence, they are referred to as essential fatty acids, the type of fats that your body needs to function properly.

Ninety-five percent of the U.S. population is deficient in EFAs Omega 3-6-9 fats, because our over-processed diets contain as much as 95% bad fats (hydrogenated oils.). If you check the processed foods in your house, you will find that almost all of them contain trans fats or partially hydrogenated vegetable oils. Dietary fat is essential for proper assimilation of certain vitamins and other nutrients. They are necessary for proper growth and are the building blocks of the prostaglandins that are essential for normal brain function. The standard North American diet lacks Omega-3 EFAs. Normally, the North American diet has about a ratio of 25:1 Omega-6 to Omega-3 EFAs. This ratio is far out of balance and should be much less excessive (3:1). Several scientific studies show that consumption of Omega-3 essential fatty acids (EFA's) leads to a substantially lower risk of death from coronary heart disease.

Eskimo natives of Greenland were studied by Danish researchers sixty years ago. Dr. H.O. Bang and scientists from the University of Alborge in Denmark observed that Eskimos consumed large amounts of fatty ocean fish which are loaded with Omega-3 oils. They were surprised to learn that of the thousands of Eskimos they investigated, only a few showed mild signs of heart disease. In fact, heart disease is so rare that Eskimos don't have a single word in their language to describe it! Researchers at Vanderbilt University studied the effects of Omega-3 on hypertension. They confirmed that Omega-3 significantly lowered high blood pressure.

Flax Seed Oil is the richest source of these EFA's. Flax seed oil contains the highest level of alpha-linolenic acid of any known plant source. These foods are not very popular in the average American diet. This deficiency plays a role in practically all degenerative diseases like heart disease and cancer, arthritis, skin conditions, diabetic neuropathy, diminished immune function and premenstrual syndrome, decreased memory and mental abilities, tingling sensation of the nerves, poor vision, increased tendency to form blood clots, increased triglycerides and "bad" cholesterol levels, impaired membrane function, hypertension, irregular heart beat, learning disorders, menopausal discomfort, and growth retardation in infants and children.

The brain is 25% fat and much of this fat is in the form of essential fatty acids. One of the most common symptoms of Omega-3 deficiency is depression, among other mental health symptoms, and of course depression is common among Americans. Low cholesterol is a risk factor for suicide. Studies show that children who have deficiencies in Omega-3 have more behavioral, learning, and health problems than do normal children. It is interesting to note that children with low levels of Omega-6 fatty acids do not have these problems. They do, however, have more colds and used antibiotics more frequently than their normal peers.

EFAs help you burn excess fat, restore health to the cardiovascular system, relieve arthritis pain and inflammation, and strengthen the immune system. A primary function of EFAs is the production of prostaglandins, which regulate body functions such as heart rate, blood pressure, blood clotting, fertility, conception, and play a role in immune function by regulating inflammation and encouraging the body to fight infection. It's important to minimize the intake of trans fats and cholesterol (animal fat) while consuming enough good fats (flaxseed oil, olive oil, ground flax seed). Flaxseed oil and gamma-linolenic (GLA) oils are referred to as the "medicinal oils." They have extensive healing properties, and minute amounts go a long way toward health. Flaxseed oil is the most abundant known source of lignans, Lignans are a special form of insoluble fiber. Flaxseed oil contains 57% Omega-3 fatty acid which is twice as much Omega-3 as fish oil. In addition, it contains only 17% linoleic acid

(Omega-6), helping to balance out the EFA ratio. Compelling studies, some funded by the National Cancer Institute, have demonstrated impressive health benefits, including positive effects in relieving hot flashes, as well as anti-cancer, antibacterial, antifungal, and antiviral activity. The anti-cancer activity may be the most promising. Flax-seed lignans are changed by human intestinal bacteria into compounds which are extremely protective against cancer, particularly breast cancer.

First things first. You should absolutely stop using all margarine and foods that have trans fats or hydrogenated oils in them. That means you are going to have to start reading a lot more and paying closer attention to the ingredients. Start using extra virgin, first cold press, olive oil as your primary oil. Smart Balance Buttery Spread is what my family uses in place of margarine. Coconut oil, peanut oil, and vegetable oils are fine if that's all you can afford. Women should take at least 1 to 2 tablespoons of flax seed oil daily. Our grandparents got these oils from the vegetables and meat they ate. However, over the past 50 years, our soils have been defiled, and most commercial farm animals eat man-made feed, which contains absolutely no essential fatty oils. The heart, brain, and immune system in particular, as well as the rest of the body, must have these oils on a regular basis in order to reverse and prevent degenerative diseases. Remove your table salt and replace it with Celtic Sea Salt. Believe it or not, salt is vitally important to overall heart health. Again your heart, brain, and immune system absolutely need the minerals and trace minerals found in real Celtic Sea Salt to function properly.

Drink plenty of distilled water and lay off the soda. Stop drinking milk and get your calcium from vegetables, raw organic almonds, and the sun. The near-vegetarian women of Papua, New Guinea, drink no milk after weaning, and have the lowest incidence of osteoporosis in the world. The body produces cholesterol and fat naturally. Refined sugar and animal fat raises cholesterol levels in the body. So as you can see, there are just too many things we are consuming, that are causing us to produce more cholesterol and fat than the body can manage at one time. Seafood and shellfish are very high in cholesterol, toxins and other heavy metals. All of these substances take a heavy toll on the heart. Parasitic worms that we maily ingest through meat consumption also attack the heart muscle and can cause all kinds of problems as they eat holes through the heart. Pork consumption has the highest concentration of such parasites. Some of these worms can lay as many as 1,000,000 eggs in a day. The easiest way to control these parasites is to use a parasitic detox program and avoid pork. Remember, most doctors do not diagnose this condition, because it is not a part of their training.

The skin of the body is really just a huge sponge that absorbs chemicals from both the water and the air. I never realized just how sensitive the skin was until I joined the United States Marine Corps, and was taught about the use of chemical and biological agents that can wipe out an entire platoon just by coming in contact with the skin. Some agents can kill in a matter of moments in very small amounts. Because the skin is so sensitive, it should be treated with extra care. A lot of lotions and perfumes contain harsh chemicals that actually poison the blood. If you can't read the ingredients, don't use it, especially if it contains hydrogenated oils. The body has to rob itself of necessary minerals in order to neutralize these toxins. Perming of the hair should be avoided because the chemicals contained in it goes right into the scalp and into the blood stream. Birth defects have been associated with hair perms.

Birth control medications adversely alter the healthy balance of intestinal flora. This leads to the overgrowth of candida yeast, which can lead to weight problems and degenerative diseases such as Type II diabetes. If you are not married, then abstinence should be your only course of action. With that said, if you are going to use birth control anyway, then it is imperative that you avoid refined sugar and products that have been processed. Candida bacteria feeds off of sugary substances and can easily grow out of control and spread to other areas of the body. Routine exercise is vitally important for a woman's health, both physically and mentally. Studies have indicated that women who exercise moderately, just 4 to 5 times per week, improve their overall health by extending their lives by an additional 15 to 20 years. Exercise also helps to reduce the severity of symptoms a woman may experience while going through PMS, menopause, and other hormonal imbalances. **Remember, God has placed before you life and death, sickness and disease, so choose life, that you and your seed may live.**

C H A P T E R 10

Scripture Misinterpretation

"I have set before you life and death, blessing and cursing: therefore choose life, that both thou and thy seed may live:" (Deuteronomy 30:19)

Misunderstanding scripture and wrong interpretation, in my opinion, is one of the major causes of unhealthy eating habits in the body of Christ today. I want to address a few of the major ones here, but before I go any further, in order to properly exegete scripture, you must first understand who it is written to and for what purpose. If one were to read the entire Bible three or four times over, they would soon realize that out of the 66 books it contains, all but 13 books and 26 chapters are written for a non-Hebrew audience. The remaining 51 books and 52 chapters are all written about Hebrew culture and history past, present and future. From Genesis, Chapter 1 to the last verse in Chapter 11, we're dealing with mankind in general. Genesis, Chapter 12, all the way through to Acts, Chapter 13, Verse 46, deals with a Hebrew audience. Acts, Chapter 14 takes us through to 2nd Thessalonians dealing with a non-Hebrew Christian audience. We have the four pastoral letters next, and from Hebrews to the book of Revelation, we are dealing with a Hebrew Christian audience. The books of Thessalonians and Revelation are both apocalyptic in nature, with the former addressing a non-Hebrew Christian audience and the latter addressing a Hebrew Christian audience.

Many people over emphasize the Gospels, even though they are very important as they are the foundation of Christianity. You must remember that Jesus never taught or preached outside the area of Palestine during His entire earthly ministry. In fact, upon sending out the first 12 disciples, He commanded that they not go the way of the Gentiles or Samaritans. So Jesus' ministry was strictly to the Jews. Matthew 10:2 "Do not go among the Gentiles or enter any towns of the Samaritans. Go rather to the lost sheep of Israel." With this in mind, we must exegete scripture from a Hebrew Christian perspective to fully grasp and understand its meaning, not in our own English language.

Today, so many people are eating and drinking everything they can get their hands on, basically because of this one scripture where Jesus declared all things clean. Mark 7:18-19 says, "Are you so dull?" he asked. "Don't you see that nothing that enters a man from the outside can make him unclean? 19) For it doesn't go into his heart but into his stomach, and then out of his body." People commonly use this one scripture as the back drop to continue in deadly generational habits that have sickened them and taken the lives of their loved ones as they helplessly stood by and watched. You hear them make comments like, "Oh! it runs in my family. Both my mother and grandmother died of diabetes." Or this is another popular one, "his father and grandfather both suffered with high blood pressure."

Yes, this one scripture has caused many people to eat themselves into early graves and a life full of unnecessary suffering. The entire conversation was not so much about food, but about unclean thoughts and motives of the heart. Verses 21-23 makes this very clear. Jesus was saying that foods cannot force a person to have thoughts of adultery, fornication, pride, or murder. In other words, if a man were to go out and sleep with his neighbor's wife, he couldn't say, "Oh, by the way, the food made me do it." So as it pertains to dealing with the human heart, all foods are clean, because they can't produce a spiritual or emotional response. However, if you were to feed your child just one serving of the deadly blow fish, they would drop dead in a matter of moments. The poisons in the blow fish would have no affect on their heart spiritually, but would stop it cold physically.

Really, one would have to study Jewish customs and culture to understand that Jews didn't consider certain foods as being edible unless it was a part of their normal dietary customs, in the same way that most people living here in America wouldn't consider monkeys, giraffes, rats, dogs, and cats as being ordinary food. These animals are not a part of our normal dietary customs, so we don't consider them as food when we envision going out to eat. John the Baptist ate wild locusts, something you and I would never recognize as food. Imagine having the whole church over for dinner after service one Sunday and serving wild locusts smothered in gravy as the main dish. You would find yourself all alone in a matter of seconds, and would never have to worry about inviting them over to eat ever again. To take this a step further, we can simply read Peter's statements to God upon waking from a vision he received in Acts, Chapter 10. In this chapter, Peter thought God was telling him to eat unclean foods when in actuality, God was preparing him for ministry to new Gentile converts. Peter vehemently exclaims in verse 14, "Surely not Lord! I have never eaten anything impure or unclean."

We can all attest to the fact that out of the 12 disciples Peter, James, and John were closest to Jesus and traveled with Him most of the time. In fact, Peter was one of the very first disciples to serve in the ministry of Jesus. These men ate, drank, slept, worked, and hung out with Jesus just like family. Even going along with Him to the top of a 9,000 foot summit where Jesus was transfigured in their presence. It is interesting then that Peter exclaims, "I have never eaten anything impure or unclean." Jesus taught and obeyed Jewish laws and customs during his ministry. His miracles and actions that caused such a controversy were an attempt to show the religious leaders that their interpretation of the law was flawed. In seeming to break the law, He was actually trying to show them how to properly interpret and apply the law.

There are two scriptures that bring this out very clearly. In Matthew, Chapter 8, Verse 1, Jesus heals the Jewish leper and then tells him to go before the priest and offer the sacrifice required by the law of Moses. However, when dealing with the Gentile Samaritan woman in John, Chapter 4, she is instructed to do just the opposite, even though in Verse 19 she is under the impression that she will have to offer up a sacrifice. While obeying Jewish laws and customs in healing the leper, Jesus followed Jewish protocol. However, with the Samaritan woman, He was actually showing her a shadow of the type of worship that would soon replace the laws of Moses. I bring this point out to show you that Jesus lived under Jewish customs even as He interacted with non-Jews. When you and I interact with foreigners today, we continue to practice our own customary traditions. Now Peter, after being around Jesus for three years and even buying food for Him, is appalled that God, knowing Jewish customs, would have the nerve to ask him to defile himself by eating unclean foods.

Peter is frightened by the thought of this to the point of becoming deeply disturbed in his spirit. Peter's disposition would indicate that the disciples never ate anything impure or unclean during their entire ministry with Jesus. In fact, there is not one scripture that speaks of Jesus eating anything unclean, and upon His resurrection, was served broiled fish with honey.

As devoted to Jesus as Peter was, had he witnessed Jesus eating anything unclean, he would not have been so offended and frightened by this vision from God. When Jesus declared all things clean, he was referring to foods that the Jews considered part of their dietary culture. This is why even now, you can't just carelessly go out and eat or touch every animal, insect, or plant you happen to stumble upon. Today, we have Campbell's Cream of Mushroom Soup as well as restaurants who serve a plethora of mushroom entrees. Mushrooms are pretty much a common food in this country and around the world. Yet, sadly, people die every year in pursuit of edible wild mushrooms. Obviously when Jesus declared all things clean, he was speaking of certain foods which God created and consecrated to be eaten.

I want to also point out the fact that the foods Jesus blessed almost 2000 years ago are not the same foods you and I eat today. Recently, restaurants and certain grocers across the nation banned the sale of a new species of fish called super fish. These fish are genetically altered with bio-engineered growth genes that make them grow eight times larger than normal fish and in just half the time. These scientifically-altered fish, to include shrimp, are able to live in cold water and not get diseases. One of the reasons why God created the Israelites was to destroy the giants in the earth in that time. Satan is always trying to counter the plans of God by producing a counterfeit. In the Old Testament, we read about how God destroyed the giants before and after the flood. There is a vivid account of one such battle in 1st Samuel 17:49 where David defeats the Philistine giant Goliath. God also used the great floods to destroy giants who defiled the earth in Noah's days.

You may ask the question, what's so wrong with giants? For one, giants require more oxygen and food to survive than people of normal height and weight. Imagine making someone angry who stands a towering 16 feet tall. Or this same person under the control and influence of Satan, with evil thoughts and intentions all the time. Satan wants to reintroduce giants back into the earth. As I stated earlier in Chapter 3 regarding the male salmon only developing female reproductive organs after being exposed to high levels of estrogen, many of our young men and woman are taller, bigger, and developing breast in their early teens. Clothing and shoe manufacturers are having to make new 3X and 4X sized apparel. The only thing that has changed in the last 30 years is the way our foods are processed and what's in them.

Whatever you eat will definitely have an impact on your body. One of the reasons why milk is associated with the development of certain types of cancer is because of the growth hormones it contains. It is also believed that these hormones can exaggerate the growth and reproduction of cancerous cells in the body. If the growth hormones forces chickens and cows to over produce, it has to have some affect on humans to a degree. The reason these food conglomerates refused to sell this new type of species is because the unknown risk to humans is so great. Scientists are warning that if these species ever escape into the wild and mate, the consequences could be disastrous for the entire world. Here again, man is being used by the evil forces in heavenly places to defile the food supply and corrupt the earth. The only thing fish farmers are concerned about is keeping their pockets lined with profits. The bigger and faster these fish grow, the more money they can make. The love of money is the root of all evil. We can barely get along with each other now. I would hate to see this world full of angry and short-tempered giants.

It is very dangerous to misinterpret scripture simply to justify one's own point of view. Look at the afflictions destroying believers today such as heart disease, cancer, diabetes, hypertension, obesity, and kidney failure which have no respect of person. They afflict the lives and rain on the just as well as the unjust. I hear people argue about wine in the Bible all the time as not being what some would consider real wine that could intoxicate an individual. Scripture clearly teaches that Noah, upon departing the ark after the flood, became drunk with wine while offering sacrifices before the Lord. Who taught Noah the proper way to offer up sacrifices in the first place? Whoever taught him must have instructed him to use the clean animals only, as stated in Genesis 8:20. He must have also been instructed about the use of wine during these ceremonies. In the same way that Adam taught his sons, Cain and Abel, how to offer up proper sacrifices before the Lord, Noah also learned from his parents and grandparents. Remember, Noah came from the righteous blood line of Seth, from which Christ would descend, which is one of the reasons why God found favor in him.

If we are going to say that it wasn't real wine that made Noah drunk, then we should also say that the animals he sacrificed weren't real either. Noah was instructed by God to bring real living clean and unclean animals aboard the ark in Genesis 7:2. Now I am not trying here to introduce a new denominational doctrine, nor am I trying to persuade you not to follow what your church teaches regarding wine. The only two religions that prohibit the consumption of wine are Islam and Buddhism. I want to make this very clear so that no one goes out and says that I am in any way propagating a new doctrine. I'm simply trying to keep it real and not reinterpret the Bible to get someone to comply with my desires. That would truly be using the scripture as a form of witchcraft. The word of God should never be used to control or enslave people. The last time I remember reading, it stated that Christ came to free us from legalism and bondage. During slavery, slave owners in this country used the Bible to justify their desire to own slaves. What's amazing is the fact that some slaves actually believed them because the master misinterpreted scripture. If you want to save your health and that of your family, you had better start searching out the truth for yourself. If the entire ship is sinking with degenerative diseases, don't just simply stand there and watch. Grab some life jackets, get your family and loved ones, and jump overboard. I'd rather take my chances swimming in an unknown ocean than to know that I am going to eventually suffer with cancer, diabetes, and heart failure if I keep hanging around.

God makes a new covenant with Noah Genesis 9:3, "everything that lives and moves shall be yours for food, just as I gave you the green plants, I now give you everything." Now immediately Verse 4 follows: "But you must not eat meat that has its lifeblood in it." Today, we know that deadly viruses can live in the blood long after death. God was actually protecting the health of Noah and his family by not allowing them to eat the blood of animals. This simple hygienic practice is currently saving countless lives around the world. Genesis 8:20 says, "Then Noah built an alter to the Lord and taking some of all the clean animals and clean birds, he sacrificed burnt offerings on it." We have already concluded that Noah learned proper sacrificial etiquette from his ancestors. Notice how Noah used the clean animals only to offer up sacrifices. These instructions had to came from God, and we see them again mentioned in the book of Leviticus, Chapter ll.

There are wild plants in nature that can cause sickness and death if ingested. Just simply touching the skin of the Amazon Dart Frog will kill you. Thousands of people around the world have died by simply tasting a teaspoon size serving of the deadly blowfish. Three hundred thousand people were sickened in China after un-knowingly eating raw contaminated clams. Some people have been permanently injured from the toxins contained in some shellfish. God never meant for humans to eat these poisonous crustaceans for our own safety. It is interesting to point out the fact that people will risk their lives eating deadly animals, but are very cautious and will avoid eating deadly plants.

If God meant for you to eat everything he blessed, then it wouldn't matter what you put into your mouth. You could bless and eat anything and everything you wanted without ever becoming sick or dying, but this has been proven not to be the case. The Bible does not contradict itself; we've simply misinterpreted it. If you are going to overcome the afflictions that are ailing you, then you must understand. God blessed everything for its divine intended purpose. You see, the poisons in the Amazon Dart Frog allow it to eat and control the population of other deadly insects. This keeps the eco-system in the jungle balanced so that other animals can live. The deadly toxins in the Blow Fish allow it to neutralize dangerous toxins in the oceans so that other species can survive. Only God could create something from matter, poison it, authorize it to live, and then ordain it to preserve creation. What a mighty and awesome God we serve. These types of species are very unique and without their help, the oceans and jungles would become unlivable, which would negative-ly impact our lives.

In the book of Acts, Peter is in a trance and sees a sheet being let down from heaven containing all kinds of four footed animals, reptiles, and birds. Verse 13 says, "Then a loud voice said get up Peter and eat." 14: "Surely not Lord! Peter replied. I have never eaten anything impure or unclean." Remember this is Peter, one of the founding fathers of Christianity, and he says emphatically, not me Lord. I have never eaten anything unclean. Peter, being Jewish, didn't consider unclean foods as part of his normal dietary customs. For example, if a friend of yours ask you to come out and try a new restaurant, you wouldn't expect to be served barbecued elephant or giraffe meat sauteed in sesame sauce and dressed with mixed vegetables. These animals are not part of your normal diet. You would expect to eat foods you are familiar with.

In this vision, God was preparing Peter for ministry to the Gentiles who were forbidden to associate with the Jews. God was letting Peter know that everyone He saves is clean. Verse19 says, "While Peter is yet pondering the vision, the Spirit said to him, three men are looking for you, don't hesitate to go with them." The three men were God-fearing Gentiles. God was using this vision to prepare Peter so that he wouldn't offend these new Gentile converts, and not so that he could defile his body with unclean foods. This is why three men showed up, and not three little pigs.

In 1st Timothy 4:3-5, Paul is dealing with the Gnostics, who believed that all matter was unclean. So they forbade marriage, sex and certain foods which God created to be received. Verse 3, says, "Forbidding to marry, and commanding to abstain from foods which God created to be received with thanksgiving by those who believe and know the truth." The word "which" references selection and is used as a restrictive clause- foods which God created to be eaten. When you are being served in a restaurant, the waiter will ask you which item from the menu you are going to select. Although there may be as many as forty items on the menu, you select which item you are going to eat. Paul is trying to convince the Gnostics that matter, which has been consecrated by the word of God, is good. Verse 4 states, "for everything God created is good, and nothing is to be rejected if it is received with thanksgiving." Verse 5, "because it is consecrated by the word of God and prayer." The word of God consecrated certain foods, which He created with specificity for human consumption for those who believe and know the truth. We don't have the inherent power to perfectly create anything. Our entire existence must be solely dependent upon God, even concerning what we should eat.

Everyone wants to believe that Jesus dying on the cross somehow changed the physical and molecular structure of both humans and animals. I'm sorry to disappoint you, but Jesus dying on the cross caused no physical changes to our bodies or that of the animals. People had the same problems controlling their fleshly desires after Christ died as they did before He died. The purpose of Christ dying on the cross was to simply restore the missing jewel of intimate worship that was lost through the fall of Adam. Remember, Satan caused a rebellion in heaven because he wanted to be worshiped. In the wilderness, he tempted Jesus and said to Him, "If you worship me, I'll give you the wealth of the earth." He has always wanted to be worshiped as if he were God and deserved it. So God created mankind strictly to worship Himself, and in the course of worship, God would personally fellowship with us.

We were created a little lower than the angels from worthless dust of the ground, then given authority over the universe that God created as a further insult to Satan. Not only are angels more intelligent than us, but they are also more powerful and stronger than we are. So the creation of mankind, then giving him dominion over the universe, was really a big slap in the face to all of the angels who rebelled with Satan.

Again, you and I were created to worship God in the beauty of his Holiness. Christ dying on the cross was to restore that lost element of man's original creation, and not to make chitterlings, fat back, and bacon edible. He died to restore lost humanity back to a right standing with God so that intimate worship could be restored. As a matter of fact, Jesus hinted this to the Samaritan woman who was converted at the well. John 4:24 says, "But the hour is coming, and now is when the true worshipers will worship the father in spirit and in truth, for the father is seeking such to worship him." The operative word here is intimate worship without the need of a priest or a human intercessor.

Today we bless our foods as if miraculously, all of the hormones, antibiotics, and parasites are going to simply walk away from our plates, as we close our eyes. When you're done praying over your food and open your eyes, the food on your plate is still just as deadly.

The only difference is you've given thanks for it. The bone and muscle meat of the chicken is still the same. Whatever was fed to that chicken during its lifetime, you are about to eat. So before you pick up that spoon and fork, ask yourself, "do I really need to defile the temple of the Holy Spirit one more day?" If you were to allow yourself to truly be led by the Spirit, He would want you to make the healthier choices. **Remember, God has placed before you life and death, sickness and disease, so choose life, that you and your seed may live.**

C H A P T E R 11

Unhealthy Generational Deadly Habits

"I have set before you life and death, blessing and cursing: therefore choose life, that both thou and thy seed may live:" (Deuteronomy 30:19)

We all carry around suitcases full of bad habits that have been passed to us over the years. One of the reasons why we eat the foods we eat is because they are part of our generational history. Actually, the main reason is that they are loaded with sugar, which masks and covers the bitter aftertaste of the poisons contaminating our food supply. Remove the sugar from your favorite yogurt, ice cream, cookies, or soda, and you wouldn't touch it. Have you ever eaten unsweetened yogurt? It doesn't taste very good. If you notice in the dairy section of the grocery store, buttermilk takes up very little space. Why? Because it's not loaded with sugar to mask the nasty taste. If buttermilk was loaded with sugar, it would take up more space on grocery store shelves. Imagine trying to drink an unsweetened soda or eat a bowl of unsweetened ice cream. I can feel you starting to hate me already. The fact is, the sugar is there purposely so that you don't taste the real poisons in the foods you eat.

For example, sodium nitrite and sodium sulfate are two deadly additives that are common in processed meats. In the human stomach, sodium nitrite is converted to nitrous acid, a mutagen (defined as a substance that causes genetic change). Sodium sulfate is added to mask the smell of rotting meat and give meat a bloody, reddish fresh look. Sodium sulfate is a poison that destroys Vitamin B, and it is capable of causing considerable damage to the digestive system and other organs. Now, if you were to pour these two additives and preservatives into a cup knowing how unhealthy they are, you wouldn't casually drink them or even think twice about giving them to your children. Yet everyday, without concern, we feed our children this unhealthy garbage and tell them to simply "bless it and eat it." You cannot feed your children unhealthy food day after day, even in small quantities and expect, over time, for it to positively affect their little bodies. After they are done saying grace, these deadly mutagen additives remain in the food. A recent study has concluded that heavy consumers of processed lunch meats have more than a 60% chance of developing colon cancer over their lifetime. The Associated Press wrote in 1994: "Children who eat more than 12 hot dogs a month develop the risk of childhood leukemia, nine times above normal." Stop forcing our children to bless and eat foods that are not blessing them. I have listed what I believe are some common generational habits that everyone should examine. If there are areas that need adjusting, then I suggest you take action immediately so that you and your seed may live in good health.

Meat

The list of diseases known to be associated with meat looks like the index of a medical textbook. Breast, colon and prostate cancer to obesity are just a few on that list. In the past few years, we've seen unprecedented recalls of meats tainted with ecoli bacteria, the outbreak of S.A.R.S, and the recent Bird Flu scare, which caused a global panic and resulted in many deaths. Take a trip through the local meat packing house in your area and see for yourself how meat is processed. The recent mad cow nightmare revealed that the brains of sick and infected cows were being mixed into cow stock feed. Most European countries have banned the import of American beef. Thirty to fifty percent of supermarket chickens are contaminated with salmonella which, you might be surprised to know can survive microwave cooking.

Over half of all antibiotics produced in this country are used just to keep animals alive long enough to get them to the slaughter houses. If the animals are too sick and unable to walk on their own, they are carried to the slaughter house by crane or forklift. In recent years, the percentage of infections resistant to penicillin went up from 15% to 85%. In fact, you may have read or heard that the McDonald's corporation recently halted the use of all super antibiotics used exclusively by their meat producers. The U.S. Center for Disease Control has concluded that antibiotics added to animal stock feed have subsequently caused animals to develop highly resistant strains of bacteria. It is estimated that 20% to 25% of all bacterial infections in the U.S. stem directly from the consumption of meats.

Try this experiment one day. Pull the plug on your freezer, or take a piece of wrapped raw meat and place it outside in the sun. Leave it alone for a week. When you open the freezer door, you will smell the stink of death. Although your freezer is air tight, you will not be in the room alone. In your freezer and in the unwrapped meat will be worms and maggots. How in the world did they get there? They were in the meat all along and you've been eating them. Did you know that the number one cause of parasitic infestation comes from the consumption of meats? These parasites nest in your eyeballs, liver, heart, lungs, intestines, brains, beneath your finger and toe nails, and other areas of your body. If you do a total parasitic cleanse and stay off meats, you will notice the darkened areas of you finger and toe nails returning to their normal color. Think for a moment, were you born with darkened finger nails and toe nails? Of course not, and you didn't have meat as part of your diet either. These parasites can cause all kinds of havoc in the body, to include symptoms of depression, as they eat away at available tissue and leave behind a toxic residue.

There is no longer any doubt about the fact that eating too much meat is a real health hazard. It is the saturated fat in the meat that does the most harm. In biblical days, fat was trimmed from all meats and was never eaten. This, of course, now makes perfect sense, and is a recommended prevention against heart disease. Trimming the fat will prevent cholesterol and triglyceride levels from rising. Most people have been brainwashed and are misinformed with regard to the amount of protein they should consume daily. Third-world nations all over the globe, who get enough calories in their diets, eat little or no meat. Yet many of them are in excellent health eating only plant protein. People who suffer kidney failure are told not to eat meat. As I said earlier, some 40 million Americans are at risk of kidney failure. Wouldn't it make sense to avoid this health problem all together, and simply lower meat consumption. Vegetable source proteins are good for us, easy to digest, and can supply all of our nutritional needs.

Large amounts of meat, dairy products and fried foods are the main cause of arteriosclerosis, coronary heart disease, stroke, certain forms of cancer, and obesity. Take a look at one of the strongest animals in the jungle, the ape, who can lift three times its own weight but eats no meat. The average person consumes over 100 grams of protein a day, and can't even lift half their own weight. We consume four to five times as much as experts now say is necessary. Do you understand why experts can't claim to have an expert science? Because they're always changing their opinion and recommendations. We all know that protein is an essential nutrient, but what most of us have not been told is that excessive amounts of indigestible protein can be hazardous to our health. Most people are totally unaware of the dangers of a high protein diet, because we have been inundated with misinformation and propaganda about protein more than any other food group. Since childhood, we have learned guidelines and information about animal protein, which were based on now out-dated and useless experiments used on rats dating back almost 100 years. These tests were funded by the meat, dairy, and egg industries, and then backed by the U.S. Government.

Today, doctors are advising people with kidney failure to eat very little or in some cases no meat. They have been very slow to inform the general public about the dangers of a high protein diet, but due to the staggering number of people with heart disease, and it being the number one killer in North America, Canada, and Europe, health experts are advising more and more heart disease patients and those with the propensity to develop heart disease, to avoid animal products because of the cholesterol, saturated fats, mucous, and lack of fiber. They are being told to consume more fruits, vegetables, and to exercise more.

Animal protein, once cooked, throws off uric acid which is highly acidic inside the body. To neutralize this condition, the body uses the available calcium in the blood first to try and handle this problem. If there is not enough calcium taken in through diet, the body will steal calcium from the bones where a majority of the body's calcium is stored. Most people will be shocked to learn that the calcium supplements they buy on store shelves have been synthetically produced in a laboratory. Your body cannot assimilate these synthetic products, because your body is not synthetic. Our bodies cannot survive off of synthetic products.

It has been interesting to observe over the years how expert opinions and official policies have changed, sometimes reluctantly, in the area of health and nutrition. Case in point, the subject of protein.

The importance of protein cannot be overstated, but too much protein or protein which cannot be digested causes many other health problems. Recent medical research has shown we should be more concerned about medical problems caused by consuming too much protein than not enough. This may shock most people trying to consume a lot of protein from animal and dairy products. Recent medical and scientific journals have reported that excess protein has been found to promote the growth of cancer cells, and contribute to liver and kidney disease, digestive problems, arthritis, gout, calcium deficiencies, and other harmful mineral imbalances. Populations that consume high-protein, animal-based diets have higher cancer rates and lower life-spans by as much as 25 to 35 years, compared to populations consuming lower protein vegetarian diets. In many cases, these individuals are living to be 100 years of age.

Scientists at Cornell University and the top advisor to the American Institute for Cancer Research, report there is a strong correlation between dietary protein intake and cancer of the breast, prostate, pancreas and colon. The director of Columbia University's Institute of Human Nutrition supports the strong evidence of a relationship between high-protein diets and cancer of the colon. Many people are addicted to meat and are frightened to death at the prospect of eating less of it. While this prospect may be frightening, the fact is, all of the meat we're consuming is slowly killing us. Listen, I'm not saying to totally give up on meat. I'm simply saying you don't need to eat so much of it. Most of us eat meat three to four times a day when in reality, we should only be eating meat once or at the most, twice a week. Adequate amounts of protein are vital to promoting cellular health and function. The major problem is too much dietary protein clogs your cells and forces the body's pH to shift from a healthy alkaline state to an unhealthy acidic state.

As I stated earlier, high levels of hydrogen atoms present in the body will decrease the amount of oxygen availability in the blood, and cause cell suffocation and damage. This process of cell degeneration will ultimately lead to degenerated new tissue being produced, tissues which are used to rebuild organs and repair the body. If your liver has damaged tissue that needs to be replaced, it will use this new degenerated tissue to patch itself. Over time, your liver will become degenerated and diseased also, which will have a domino affect on the body's other vital organs. As you can clearly see, it is impossible for the body to heal itself in this extended state of oxygen depletion, and taking medications won't solve the problem either. Now I want you to clearly understand the fact that all medications are toxic and acidic in the body. Putting one acidic condition on top of another does not help the problem get better, but only makes it worst. Before long, you'll have to take another medication to counteract the harmful side affects caused by the original medicine you took to treat the problem in the first place. You need oxygen to survive, not medicine. In fact, if you took medicine and didn't have oxygen, you would die. You must oxygenate your body by switching to an alkaline-producing diet so that the body can heal and repair itself, and you won't need to continuously take medications.

Seafood And Crustaceans

Seafood has become America's favorite past time, and for the first time in the history of our nation, shrimp, has now surpassed hot dogs as the number one food in this country. The majority of the shrimp consumed in this country are not from the open ocean, but rather from shrimp farms where they are bred and harvested strictly for commercial consumption. The difference between shrimp caught in the wild and those grown on farms is the quality and safety of the shrimp. The shrimp from the farms are fed pelletized food, similar to what you would feed to your pet fish. Now your pet fish will not be going to the supermarket to be sold for someone's dinner table, so the pellets you are feeding it are okay as long as the fish remains your pet. However, the pellets fed to the farmed shrimp are also mixed with antibiotics. This is where the health problem lies. These antibiotics keep the shrimp alive long enough to get them to the food processing companies. Without these antibiotics, these shrimp would die because of the toxic environment in which they are kept all of their lives. These farms are enclosed areas to quarantine the shrimp, preventing escape and stopping other species from infiltrating and eating or contaminating this precious commodity.

Most of our commercial fish are also harvested in the same way. A recent Canadian study found that a single serving of farmed salmon contains three to six times the World Health Organization's recommended daily intake limit for dioxins and PCBs. A salmon farm of 200,000 fish releases an amount of nitrogen, phosphorus, and fecal matter roughly equivalent to the nutrient waste in untreated sewage from 20,000 to 25,000 people. These fish live in this environment their entire lives without ever getting out in the wild to exercise or eat naturally occurring nutrient rich oceanic foods. Fish stay healthy by getting exercise when swimming with and against the strong currents in ocean waters, as well as by breathing fresh oxygen, unlike the air quality inside a fish farm. In the farm, these creatures eat, breathe, and swim in toxic, fecal polluted water. In fact, the biotechnology food company Monsanto has created a colored dye that is sprayed on the meat to give it a pinkish, fresh-looking texture.

Shrimp are part of the shellfish family who are bottom feeders by nature, and were created by God to help keep the ecosystem of the oceans clean and livable. They clean and filter the oceans by removing toxic waste and pollution. Shrimp, who are already toxic by nature, now become gravely toxic and are very rich in artery-clogging cholesterol. God made the bottom fish to have skin but no scales, even though many have fins. Species, such as halibut, flounder, octopus, lingcod, and catfish all have skin but no scales. Shrimp, lobster, scallops, crabs, oysters, claims, snails, and sea cucumbers all feed off the junk on the bottom of the sea and are unclean. Studies have revealed that pork and shellfish contain moderate amounts of cholesterol, toxins, and contaminates associated with human poisoning. In 1998, 300,000 people were sickened in China after eating raw, contaminated shellfish. Poisoning associated with shellfish is the number one cause of emergency hospital visits in this country. Thousands of people continue to die every year around the world after consuming raw shellfish.

Large fish, like tuna and shark, have skin and fins, but no scales. Because of their size and their ability to reach deeper waters, they have higher concentrations of heavy metals such as mercury. The medical community has been warning us for the past couple of years about the dangers of over consuming these types of fish. Smaller fish with fins and scales mostly feed near or just below the water's surface, and they filter small amounts of toxins through their gills. Their scales protect them from absorbing most toxins so they are considered clean. Some believers believe the New Testament abolished the clean and unclean laws mentioned in the book of Leviticus. However, the clear distinction between clean and unclean predates the laws given to Moses at Mt. Sinai. Noah was instructed by God himself to bring clean and unclean animals aboard the ark long before the nation of Israel ever existed.

The next time you sit down to enjoy a platter full of seafood, consider this. These crustaceans live their entire lives transforming our oceans into clean, livable environments. The dangerous toxins they remove from the waters stays eternally locked-up in the muscle meet of their bodies throughout their lives. This explains why they are hard shelled creatures, to prevent re-contamination. Have you ever opened a crab, clam, or lobster and noticed all of the nasty, gooey stuff surrounding the meat. You guessed it, disgusting and highly toxic feces is what you are staring at and have your hands all in. What's even more amazing is some people actually eat the feces as a delicacy. There are several scriptures in the Bible that speak of God being offended by the presence of fecal matter. Now if God doesn't want it around him, He definitely doesn't want us to defile the temple of the Holy Spirit with it. The crustaceans role is to keep the oceans clean of toxins, not add extra pollutants to it. God loves us so much, that He decided to protect us by creating these creatures with a hardened outer shell. The foreign toxins you ingest will start to defile and poison your blood, which again is the life of the all flesh. So they are placed in the oceans to protect us and the environment, not for our dinner tables. People who have elevated cholesterol or heart trouble are told by their doctors to avoid seafood.

Table Salt vs. Celtic Sea Salt

When one speaks of salt, they must make a clear distinction between mineral-depleted refined table salt and real unrefined grey mineral-rich Celtic Sea Salt. Table salt should be avoided at all costs, because it is totally unhealthy and dangerous to your health. It should be replaced instead with Celtic Sea Salt. The Celtic word for salt is "holy" or "sacred." In the Bible, salt symbolizes a vital part of God's covenant with His people: "<u>And every oblation of thy meat offering shalt thou season with salt; neither shalt thou suffer the salt of the covenant of thy God to be lacking from thy meat offering: with all thine offerings thou shalt offer salt.</u>" Leviticus 2:13. Elisha purified a spring by casting salt into it (2nd Kings 2:19-22). In the Sermon on the Mount, Jesus referred to his disciples as "the salt of the earth" (Matt.

5:13). From the beginning of history, salt was exalted and synonymous with virtue. Salt was so precious that spilling it was considered a bad omen. Entire civilizations were built and financed from salt revenues including the great wall of China.

The chemical and mineral compositions of our blood have an amazing similarity to salty sea water. Our tears, blood, and sweat taste much like it. Before God created dry land, oceans covered the earth Genesis 1:9. Genesis 2:7 says "The Lord God formed man from the dust of the ground." So our bodies are made of dust (dry land) and seawater. Our bodies contain three internal oceans that require a regular replenishment of minerals and trace elements. One of these oceans forms the plasma of our blood, another the lymphatic circulatory system, and last, the extracellular fluid. Every living cell is bathed in a mineral-rich regenerating solution called extracellular fluid. These three internal oceans are interconnected, greatly influencing each other, and are amazingly similar to the composition of sea water.

The same 87 mineral elements found in our bodies are contained in sea water. It is impossible for the body to function without salt. Salt stabilizes irregular heartbeats, regulates blood pressure, and extracts excess acidity from the brain cells. It balances sugar levels in the blood and is vitally needed to treat diabetics. It facilitates cells' communication and information processing from the moment of conception to death. It aids with the absorption of food particles through the intestinal tract. It is vital for the clearance of mucus and sticky phlegm from the lungs, particularly in people with asthma and cystic fibrosis. Salt is vital for clearing sinuses, preventing muscle cramps, firming bones, teeth, and prevents osteoporosis. It works to regulate sleep as a natural hypnotic, also preventing gout, arthritis, varicose veins, and it stops dry coughs.

A human embryo spends the first nine months of life floating in a miniature ocean inside the mother's womb. In this salty environment of amniotic fluid, it grows over 3 billion times its weight. At no time in our entire existence, from the moment we take our first breath until we breathe our last, are we ever without the need of minerals from real salt. Modern science has determined that 24 of these elements are essential for life, although a proper balance of all 87 elements in our bodies are necessary for optimum health. Herds of elephants will risk injury and death trying to reach hidden salt caves where they supplement their sodium-deficient diets. Our domesticated pets also suffer from mineral deficiencies. Table salt only has two minerals, sodium and chlorine which are poisonous, dangerous, and very deadly. Bathing in seawater has an immediate strengthening effect on the lymphatic system. Oppositely, bathing in tap water, rivers and lakes which are unsalted, mineral depleted, and some- times chlorinated, will weaken the lymph system and also drain the body's precious minerals from the other two fluids.

Celtic Sea Salt contains the same 87 minerals that make up the structure of our bodies, and is untouched by damaging refine- ment and industrial processing. Isn't it interesting that both salt and water are the only two non-biological elements that all humans and animals must have or they will die. In the book of Exodus, we learn that God provided the children of Israel with water as they wander- ed for 40 years through a salty environment. Sodium is so impor- tant, in fact, that humans have a specific sensor on the tongue that can detect salt. Violent prisoners given Celtic Sea Salt in their diets showed improved behaviors within a few short weeks. Doctors pre- scribe lithium to treat manic depressives and bipolar individuals; how- ever, the side effects of this medication can be nasty. Celtic Sea Salt contains natural lithium salts. Unlike supplementing with medicinal lithium, the lithium in Celtic Sea Salt is absorbed naturally, in quan- tities nature intended and unrefined by man.

The composition of crystal ocean salt is so complicated that no laboratory in the world can reproduce it from its basic 80 che- mical elements. Nature is still a better chemist than the medical and scientific community. No pill supplementation can equal the wealth of minerals that natural sea salt supplies, regardless of how rich or precisely that supplementation is formulated. In fact, during World War II, Navy doctors would use sea salt water for blood transfusions when blood supplies ran out. Many lives were saved.

We have been grossly mislead by the medical community when they informed us to reduce salt or take it completely out of our diets. The only problem here is that all the medical research has been based on using refined table salt only, not mineral-rich Celtic Sea Salt. If salt was so bad, why are patients in hospitals fed intravenous saline solutions? The answer is simply because the human body runs on salt. Without salt, the body runs out of electrolytes, and just like a battery, cannot run without it. The human body will die out if there are no electrolytes present. In the 1900's, a medical doctor named Jacques Loeb from the University of California, performed an epic experiment. He put fish in a tank of water mixed with refined salt, the same concentration of salt that exists in sea water, and all the fish died. If fish can't live on pure sodium chloride in dilute concentrations, neither can we.

With the natural balance of 85 or so minerals missing, the salt becomes totally useless. This is why table salt causes high blood pressure, because it is out of balance and lacks the minerals needed to regulate blood pressure. Magnesium scarcity is the cause of many diseases. Magnesium is one of the major components of all living matter. Magnesium salts are needed to stimulate white blood cell activity. They also promote the action of vitamins, and play an important role in glucose metabolism and proper calcium metabolism. Today most of what we consume, like vegetables, fruits, and grains are depleted of magnesium because of chemical fertilizers or sprayed fields.

Junk foods, such as white bread, refined sugar, and refined grain products are stripped of magnesium through refinement. Refining whole wheat and polishing rice can reduce their magnesium content. Magnesium salts, while quite abundant in young adults, become depleted in older persons. Factors affecting absorption of magnesium are: physiological need, the amount of magnesium ingested, and the diet as a whole. I have actually given Celtic Sea Salt to countless people suffering with high blood pressure without any adverse side affects. As a matter of fact, their blood pressure actually dropped overall to normal levels without the further need of medications.

Celtic Sea Salt is full of complex minerals and bio-electronic power offering countless health benefits like balancing the body's pH levels, relieving skin diseases, allergies, and restoring good digestion. It has the amazing power to reverse and heal many chronic illnesses and restore wholeness in a matter of a few days. I was once suffering with severe kidney failure after removing salt totally from my diet. I was just as clueless as the rest of the country, and followed the medical community's advice regarding salt-free diets especially for minorities and African Americans. Because of my vegetarian life-style, my diet was very rich in potassium from the dark green vegetables and certain fruits and nuts I consumed. I was on a sodium free diet, so my kidneys had to work extra hard to neutralize the potassium and flush it out of my body. This constant overworking of my kidneys started to wear them down and I developed the early signs of painful kidney failure.

Once I reintroduced Celtic Sea Salt back into my diet, within a few days, the crippling pain had totally cleared up, and I could once again bend over and touch my toes. I also took daily doses of garlic and ginseng which helped my immune system fight off the disease. Amazingly, the problem has never returned and I didn't have to see a doctor or use any costly medications. Notice how I said I used mineral-rich Celtic Sea Salt and not regular deadly table salt which only contains two minerals, sodium and chloride.

Sodium is highly explosive and will ignite when it touches water. This is why the roads are salted during snow storms. The sodium, when coming into contact with the snow, produces heat which melts it away. The chlorine is used to clean the water in our swimming pools, municipal water treatment plants, and whiten clothing. Commercial refined salt is not only stripped of all its minerals, besides sodium and chloride, but it also is heated to temperatures so high that the chemical structure of salt changes. In addition, it is chemically cleaned, bleached, and treated with anti-caking agents to remove the moisture which is caused by the presence of magnesium.

This process prevents salt from clumping up and sticking together so it shakes freely out the bottle. Unfortunately, the anti-caking agents perform the same function in the human body, so refined salt does not dissolve and combine with the water and fluids present in our system. Instead, it builds up in the body and leaves deposits in the organs and tissues as cellulite causing severe health problems. Two of the most common anti-caking agents used in the mass production of salt are sodium aluminum silicate and aluminum calcium silicate. Both are sources of aluminum, a toxic metal that has been implicated in the development of Alzheimer's disease. These toxins certainly don't belong in a healthy diet. To make matters worse, the aluminum used in salt production leaves a bitter taste in salt, so manufacturers usually add sugar in the form of dextrose to hide the caustic taste of aluminum. Refined sugar severely disrupts the equilibrium of the body and is associated with the development of more than 130 diseases.

Whether you consider the unbalanced mineral condition of the salt we use, the anti-caking agents that prevent salt from doing some of its most important jobs in the body, or the chemicals and sugar that are added to it, table salt should be avoided because it is, without a doubt, hazardous to human health. Table salt makes the body highly acidic, prohibits digestion leading to malnutrition, which in my opinion is a major cause of disease in this country. When commercially-processed American foods, full of refined salt, arrived in Africa, something hardly ever seen before arrived with it- cancer. In countries which do not alter their supply of salt, heart disease and arthritis are so rare that many doctors have never seen a case. Sodium is an essential nutrient which the body cannot produce, but is required for life and good health. Life begins with electrolytes. Trace minerals carry the life force in our bodies more than any other substance. Mineral salts create electrolytes. Electrolytes, often called the spark of life, are what carry the electrical currents throughout our bodies, sending messages to the cells in all of the different systems. Electrolytes are also necessary for enzyme production. Enzymes are responsible for breaking down food, for absorbing nutrients, muscle function, hormone production and more.

Celtic sea salt strongly alkalinizes the body, making it a strong and powerful remedy. In all of the following conditions– acute infection, severe burns, hemorrhaging, deep emotional turmoil, physical trauma, or shock from illness or surgical intervention– extra potassium is immediately required by the body. The potassium will be replenished quickly through the process of transforming sodium to potassium. The concentration of salt diminishes in the blood as sodium transforms into potassium.

Biologically, we need natural-occurring minerals and trace minerals from salt to maintain optimum cellular function. These minerals must be replenished regularly on a daily basis, and are necessary and vital for every bodily function. Many common illnesses and poor health conditions have been traced to a deficiency of minerals. Ironically, the minerals are found in sea salt. The problem is that common table salt has lost its savor and is no longer good for the body. Luke 14:34-35 says "salt is good, but if the salt has lost its savor, wherewith shall it be seasoned? It is neither fit for land , nor yet for the dunghill, but men cast it out."

When table salt enters the body, the body becomes toxic. In order to survive in this environment, every cell in the body wraps itself in a cocoon of water for protection. Imagine enlarged water enclosed cells now trying to squeeze and maneuver their way through blood vessels and arteries that are clogged with fat, cholesterol and plaque. Blood flow becomes severely restricted, which causes your blood pressure to rise, eventually causing a stroke or heart disease. Combine this condition of poor circulation with obesity, when the heart is forced to pump harder, and you have a deadly combination. Without the other 85 minerals, our nervous system and brain will not function properly. Without salt, our bodies cannot make adequate amounts of stomach acid. With low levels of stomach acid, our digestion is impaired and we cannot absorb minerals. Minerals are needed to activate enzymes which aid absorption of minerals for cell reproduction. This is why taking antacids is so damaging. It inhibits acid production, which then leads to disease.

Refined salt deposits into the fatty tissue and turns into cellulite. It's amazing. Everyone rich and poor, white and black, short and tall, fat and skinny, crave salt. Salt craving is always a sign of trace mineral lack. People today are starving for minerals that have been removed from both the soil and the salt. The heart muscle works harder on a low-salt diet. A salt-free diet can cause kidney, respiratory, and blood sugar problems. Only about five percent of the world's annual salt production ends up as seasoning at the dinner table. The vast majority, however, pours into chemical plants, where it leads the five major raw materials utilized by industry: salt, sulfur, limestone, coal and petroleum. Salt pickles cucumbers, helps pack meat, cans vegetables, cures leather, makes glass, bread, butter, cheese, rubber and wood pulp.

Salt has some 14,000 uses, more than any other mineral. Ninety-five percent of the sea salt goes to chemical laboratories and manufacturing companies who make most of their profits by pulling out the minerals in salt, and selling them back to us in the form of vitamins and supplements to the tune of $19 billion in annual sales. Also, companies like Kellogg's take a healthy natural food, refine and processes it until it's worthless, and then add back some fortified vitamins and minerals. These minerals come from the salt companies in the form of "fortified" foods; for example, cereals fortified with vitamins and minerals. These synthetic supplements are mineral-deficient themselves, and are not readily metabolized in our bodies. Trace minerals can be harmful if taken artificially in large doses.

In 1923, processors began refining salt. During the refining process, essential minerals were removed or altered. Shortly after salt started being refined, mental illness increased dramatically. The minerals removed from the salt are sold to make anti-knock petroleum additives, chemical fertilizers, light metal alloys, explosives, and plastics. Celtic Sea Salt is the brand of salt I recommend most often. Contrary to popular belief, removing hazardous salt out of your diet and maintaining your intake isn't as simple as putting down the salt shaker. In fact, if you're the average American, throwing away your salt shaker will hardly make a dent in your sodium intake, because salt added at the table is small compared to the salt that is hidden in processed foods we consume daily. Salt is added so insidiously and so often by the food manufacturers that it is difficult to escape it.

Salted snack foods like chips, pretzels, roasted party nuts, soups, and breads are all salted. Salt is even hidden in cereals like Corn Flakes, Pop Tarts, Frosted Flakes, cakes, pies, sodas, Sunny Delight, and even Gatorade. No matter where you purchase your food, you need to pay close attention to what's in it. Don't forget the fact that the majority of the salt Americans consume is contained in processed foods. This means you have to watch every food you think about buying and putting into your mouth. One of the best ways to limit your sodium intake is to carefully read the labels. Read the amount of sodium milligrams listed on the label of the food you consider purchasing. Although sodium needs differ for each person, as a rule of thumb, try buying low-sodium foods. Foods that have 140 milligrams or less of sodium per serving should be your standard. If additional sodium in your diet is needed, add extra salt to your meals. The use of salt is so widespread in the cooking and processing of foods that removing the salt clearly requires several different approaches. It means becoming salt smart, learning where salt normally is found, and how to do without it. It is also important to remember that the proper salt, when used in moderation either as an ingredient in cooking or added at the table, is not a problem.

To begin with, sodium is crucial for maintaining the health of every cell in the human system. Potassium and sodium are required for the proper functioning of our nerves and the contraction of our muscles. Lastly, sodium is needed to maintain several kinds of equilibrium: electrolyte balance, fluid balance, and pH balance, which are all vitally important to the body. Obtaining adequate amounts of easily absorbable sodium from the foods we eat then is important for maintaining health. However, obtaining too much of the wrong kinds of sodium or table salt is harmful. Today, sodium is often misunderstood by the public just like fat. Sodium and fat are necessary nutrients we need for optimum health, but not all forms of sodium and fat are good for us. Today, we are warned over and over again about the dangers of too much sodium intake. Excessive salt consumption causes the development of high blood pressure, but can also be associated with strokes, fluid retention, calcium deficiency, osteoporosis, weight gain, stomach ulcers and stomach cancer.

However, low or no sodium intake can be just as dangerous as too much of it. Too little can cause poor heart rhythms, increase the risk of heart attack in hypertensive patients, spasms, and sudden death. Knowing the role sodium plays in the body and the difference between "healthy" and "unhealthy" sources of sodium, will help you get the salt out of your diet while you still meet your sodium needs. The average American's salt intake is two to three teaspoons a day. This equals about 4,000 to 6,000 milligrams of sodium a day, which is double the Food and Drug Administration's maximum recommended daily allowance of 2,400 milligrams. No other mammal eats this much salt and no other mammal has the health problems we do. High blood pressure, for example, was never even seen in animals until researchers found they could induce it either by surgery or by introducing large amounts of salt into animals' diets. We unknowingly absorb excessive salt not only from the food we consume, but also from an unsuspected source, the salt-softened water in which we bathe in. The American Heart Association now warns that salt-softened water can cause elevated sodium levels, and now health-conscious Americans can no longer drink salt-softened water. Few of us, however, realize that we receive a lot of unwanted sodium every time we take a shower, a bath, or wash clothes in softened water.

Sodium absorbed through the skin and topically ingested salt has become the main reason of excess sodium. The sodium we consume from food and water is only part of the problem. The highly refined nature of common table salt is the other part. Our bodies were not designed to tolerate large amounts of sodium; however, healthy individuals usually can tolerate some excess sodium as long as it's naturally occurring in a form that our bodies can readily use or excrete. However, there are alternatives to commercial table salt. Unrefined Celtic Sea Salt is good, and the body can use many of the roles sodium can play. Celtic Sea Salt harvested off the pristine shores of Brittany, France, is a pollutant-free salt. It is not altered with coloring, additives or bleaching and it is not kiln dried. It also has a full complement of trace minerals including iodine. For all these reasons, it is a very good source of natural occurring minerals. I have listed almost 80 minerals and trace minerals needed in order for the body to function as it was designed to, both mentally and physically.

8 7 Elements Essential For Life

Of the more than 80 minerals and trace minerals that are removed from real sea salt, 75 are listed below and then resold in dangerously unbalanced concentrations. Jesus said that our conversation should be salted with peace. With all the these necessary minerals missing from our diets daily, one can clearly see why there is so much psychological and physical dysfunction in this country.

Name	Chem Sym	Name	Chem Sym
1. Aluminum	AL	2. Europium	EU
3. Molybdenum	MO	4. Fluoride	F
5. Antimony	SB	6. Strontium	SR
7. Neodymium	ND	8. Gadolinium	G.D.
9. Arsenic	AS	10. Sulfur (sulfate)	S
11. Nickel	NI	12. Gallium	GA
13. Barium	BA	14. Tantalum	TA
15. Niobium	NB	16. Germanium	GE
17. Beryllium	BE	18. Tellurium	TE
19. Osmium	OS	20. Gold	AU
21. Bismuth	BI	22. Terbium	TB
23. Palladium	PD	24. Hafnium	HF
25. Boron	B	26. Hafnium	HF
27. Phosphorus	P	28. Thallium	TL
29. Bromine	BR	30. Holmium	HO
31. Platinum	PT	32. Thorium	TH
33. Cadmium	CD	34. Indium	IN

Name	Chem Sym	Name	Chem Sym l
35. Potassium	K	36. Thulium	TM
37. Calcium	CA	38. Iodine	I
39. Praseodymium	PR	40. Tin	SN
41. Carbon	C	42. Iridium	IR
43. Rhenium	RE	44. Titanium	TI
45. Cerium	CE	46. Iron	FE
47. Rhodium	RH	48.Tungsten	W
49. Cesium	CS	50. Lanthanum	LA
51. Rubidium	RB	52. Vanadium	V
53. Ruthenium	RU	54. Lead	PB
55. Chromium	CR	56.Ytterbium	YB
57. Samarium	SM	58. Lithium	LI
59. Cobalt	CO	60.Yttrium	Y
61. Scandium	SC	62. Lutetium	LU
63. Copper	CU	64. Zinc	ZN
65. Selenium	SE	66. Magnesium	MG
67. Dysprosium	DY	68. Zirconium	ZR
69. Silico	SI	70. Manganes	MN
71. Erbium	ER	72. Oxygen	O
73. Silver	AG	74. Mercury	HG
75. Hydrogen	H		

Although certain body processes are attributed to certain minerals, each mineral needs one or more other minerals to properly function. For instance, a proper calcium-phosphorus balance is necessary to the body in that an imbalance reduces resistance to disease, increases fatigue, weakens intellectual faculties and leads to premature aging. Magnesium can only be used if calcium and phosphorus are in a proper balance. An overabundance of one mineral can result in a deficiency of another. Obtaining minerals from whole food sources provides the body with the wide variety of minerals it needs. Supplementing with one or two minerals is rarely a good idea unless it is under the supervision of a doctor or nutritional counselor.

Chloride: along with sodium, regulates the acid/alkali balance in the body. It is also necessary for the production of gastric acid which is a component of hydrochloric acid for all digestion.

Sodium: regulates the pH of intracellular fluids and with potassium, regulates the acid/ alkali balance in the body. Sodium and chloride are necessary for maintaining osmosis and electrolyte balance.

Sulfur: is found in all cells, especially in skin, connective tissues and hair. Inadequate dietary sulfur has been associated with skin and nail diseases. Increased intake of dietary sulfur sometimes helps psoriasis and rheumatic conditions.

Magnesium: is a mineral of primary importance in the body because it aids in the activation of adenosine triphosphate (ATP), the main energy source for cell functioning. Magnesium also activates several enzyme systems and is important for the synthesis of RNA and DNA. Magnesium is necessary for normal muscle contraction and important for the synthesis of several amino acids.

Potassium: exists primarily in intracellular fluids (the fluid inside cells). Potassium stimulates nerve impulses and muscle contractions and is important for the maintenance of osmotic pressure. Potassium regulates the body's acid-alkali balance, stimulates kidney and adrenal functioning, and assists in converting glucose to glycogen. Potassium is important for biosynthesis of protein.

Calcium: is necessary to build healthy bones and teeth. Calcium influences blood coagulation, stimulates muscles and nerves, and acts as a cofactor for vitamin D and the function of the parathyroid gland. Muscles cannot contract without calcium. Calcium is essential for the regulation of your heartbeat. Calcium depletion can result in a number of symptoms, the most notable is osteoporosis which results in decreased bone mass and increased chances of bone breakage.

Silicon: is necessary for normal growth and bone formation. With calcium, silicon is a contributing factor in good skeletal integrity. Silicon is a main component of osteoblasts, the bone forming cells. Silicon may help to maintain youthful skin, hair and nails.

Copper: facilitates in the absorption of iron and supports vitamin C absorption. Copper is also involved in protein synthesis and an important factor in the production of RNA.

Tin: small amounts of tin appear to be necessary for normal growth. Because tin is common in soil, foods, and water, deficiencies are rare. Because of poor absorption, low tissue accumulation and rapid tissue turnover, tin has a low level of toxicity.

Manganese: is essential for glucose utilization, for lipid synthesis and for lipid metabolism. Manganese plays a role in cholesterol metabolism and pancreatic function and development. Manganese in involved in normal skeletal growth and it activates enzyme functions.

Iron: only trace amounts of iron are essential for living cells of plants and animals. Iron has the ability to interact reversibly with oxygen, and to function in electron transfer reactions that makes it biologically indispensable. Iron is necessary for cell function and blood utilization. Blood loss is the most common cause of iron deficiency. Pallor and extreme fatigue are the symptoms of iron deficiency (anemia).

Aluminum: a natural component of many foods. Although it is found in small quantities in plant and animal tissues and in blood and urine, there is no evidence that this element is essential for any metabolic function in humans or animals. In fact, there is evidence that elevated aluminum can result in neurological disorders, bone disease, gastrointestinal irritation, loss of appetite and loss of energy. Because aluminum is a natural constituent of some foods and is in a growing number of modern foods and pharmaceutical preparations, an understanding of aluminum and aluminum-containing foods and cooking utensils can benefit all people. In healthy people, more than 98% of the ingested aluminum is passed through the gastrointestinal tract. Silicon, a constituent of Celtic Sea Salt (see above), prevents the absorption of aluminum and actually helps the body eliminate aluminum that is bound in the tissues.

Strontium: (not Strontium 90, the radioactive form of the element) may help harden the calcium-magnesium-phosphorus structures of the body. Strontium may influence the intake or structural use of calcium, according to Bernard Jensen, Ph.D.

Zinc: although adults only require an average of 15 mg of zinc per day, zinc is a very important trace element that is essential to many biological factors. Zinc is required for growth, for immune system function, and for sexual development. Zinc is a cofactor in over 90 enzymes. Zinc is required for the synthesis of insulin. Proper zinc metabolism is needed for wound healing, and carbohydrate and protein metabolism. Zinc is considered an antibacterial factor in the prostatic fluid, and may contribute to the prevention of chronic bacterial prostatitis and urinary tract infections.

Gallium: has no known biological role, although it may stimulate metabolism. Small concentrations of gallium are normally found in human tissue.

Titanium: is an abundant mineral, yet it appears to have no function to plant and animal life. In general, humans may eat and excrete titanium with no side effects as it is considered essentially nontoxic. Titanium may be carcinogenic, but not at the levels humans are generally exposed to.

Fluoride: has a direct effect on the calcium and phosphate metabolism and in small amounts, may reduce osteoporosis. Trace amounts of fluoride produce stronger tooth enamel that is more resistant to bacterial degradation. However, an increased intake through fluoridated drinking water can potentially overload the human system.

Rubidium: has a close physiochemical relationship to potassium. In fact, it may have the ability to act as a nutritional substitute for potassium. Although rubidium is not considered "essential," some evidence suggests that rubidium may have a role in free radical pathology and serve as a mineral transporter across defective cell membranes, especially in cells associated with aging. Clinical studies have suggested that rubidium increases memory and mental acuity in the elderly.

Refined White Sugar

White sugar is an unnatural substance not found anywhere in nature. After all of the vitamins, minerals, and proteins are stripped away by industrial processes, what remains is a concentrated chemical which poisons and slowly destroys the human body. Sugar has been implicated in causing over 130 known diseases, and even creating new ones as the body goes through metaphysical changes trying to handle this deadly toxin. Before I go any further, I'm sure as you read this section you'll be able to match the name of someone you know with one of the illnesses mentioned: cancer, obesity, diabetes, high cholesterol, hyperactivity, colds, anxiety, tooth decay, poor vision, gallstones, arthritis, migraine headaches, allergies, and skin eruptions. These are just a few and I'm sure as you were reading the list, you thought about many of your friends, relatives, co-workers and church members. Sugar causes your food to spoil in your stomach and also makes the process of digestion more difficult.

Sugar is highly addictive. The average American now consumes approximately 130 pounds of sugar per year compared to just 2.5 pounds 100 years ago. As far back as 1929, Dr. F.G. Banting, the discoverer of insulin, noted that the increase of diabetes in the United States was increasing proportionately with the per capita consumption of cane sugar. Sugar does more damage than any other poison, drug, or narcotic. Why? Because it is considered a food, and the damaging affects begin very early in life. Infants are introduced to this deadly chemical just hours after they are born. Almost 95% of all people are addicted to it to some degree or other.

Even though sugar has been around in minute quantities for several thousand years, it formed an insignificant part of the average diet in the civilizations of ancient Egypt, Greece, and Rome. It is interesting to note a scripture that speaks of Moses being in good health and having perfect eyesight at the age of 120. Remember, he had to hike through the plains of Moab, and then climb the mountain of Nebo to the top of Mt. Pisgah. Moses did all this at the age of 120, which indicates that he was physically fit to live even longer had God not decided to take his life. Since sugar wasn't normally consumed every day in the diets of ancient civilizations, and there were no refineries, we can conclude that refined sugar was one food Moses didn't consume. The Greeks, who had a word for nearly everything, had no word for sugar in their language.

Sugar cane was grown on Spanish soil after the Moors invaded and colonized southern Spain and started refining it. Spain inherited some of the sugar plantations when it finally drove out the Moors. This is when the Christian world first tasted this forbidden substance and became addicted. Sugar is highly addictive and tasteful, and the sweet enjoyable taste masks the deadly poison. It only takes just one taste and it becomes habit forming. A strong, insatiable craving and powerful taste develops for sugar so that people can never seem to get enough of this poison. Sugar is an unnatural chemical the body has no way of coping with. Sugar is just as harmful and deadly as heroin, and both are arrived at through similar processes of refinement. In producing heroin, the opium is first extracted from the poppy. The opium is then refined into morphine, and the morphine is further refined into heroin. Similarly, sugar is processed by first extracting juice from the cane or beet and then it's refined into molasses. Then it's further refined into brown sugar, and the end product is strange white crystals that are foreign to the human body. By the way, brown sugar is nothing more than refined white sugar sprayed with molasses. Sugar takes a long and fortunately slow and insidious time to totally ravage and destroy your body. Sugar, over time, destroys your bones, joints, and teeth by leaching vital minerals from these areas. It suppresses your immune system for extended periods of time disabling the body's ability to fight off disease. It ruins the adrenal glands, pancreas, and puts your entire endocrine system out of balance, producing an incredibly long list of damages.

American processed foods contain the most sugar of any other country on the entire earth. Everything we eat is loaded with sugar, from cereals, bread, soups, luncheon meats, crackers, and just about all processed junk foods. Some cereals touted as healthy are as much as 50% sugar. Sugar causes more damage to the human body than any other drug or narcotic, and is also a long-term chemical poison. Recently the state of Arkansas, after receiving so much pressure from mothers on PTA boards, decided to remove all junk food vending machines from their schools. During a state-wide study, officials learned that 60% of the state's children were overweight or obese. Recent studies have shown that an alarming number of obese children are starting to develop signs of diabetes.

Your body changes sugar into two to five times more fat in the blood stream than it does starches. Sugar causes hyperactivity in some children causing them to bounce of the walls as they say. Sugar given to premature babies can actually affect the amount of carbon dioxide they produce. Sugar can make the symptoms of attention deficit disorder more aggravated. Sugar and sugary drinks dehydrate the body. Patients in intensive care live longer when sugar intake is limited. Antisocial behavioral disorders were dropped by almost 50% when juveniles in rehabilitation camps were put on a low sugar diet. Sugar has been attributed to high blood pressure in obese people. Too much sugar can increase epileptic seizures and increases the risk of polio. Sugar can cut off oxygen to the brain through intravenous feeding and promote chronic degenerative diseases. A decrease in sugar intake can greatly improve emotional stability. Sugar increases the amount of free radicals in the body leading to premature aging and loss of joint elasticity. Sugar causes hormonal imbalances in both men and women, increasing estrogen in men, and complicating PMS in women. Sugar can cause depression and alter the ability to think clearly.

Sugar is definitely the number one enemy of a bowel movement. Just try this test one day and you will be totally convinced, plus you'll save money on toilet tissue. For four to five days, don't eat or drink anything with sugar in it. Increase your intake of raw, dark green leafy vegetables like broccoli, cabbage, cucumbers, spinach, mixed green salad, raw seeds or almonds, extra virgin olive oil, and green granny apples. You will notice that not only will you have a bowel movement more often, but you won't hardly need to use any toilet tissue if you use any at all. Animals in the wild don't have runny sticky stools, unlike domesticated pets who suffer with this problem when sugar is added to their diets. Sugar intake is higher in people with Parkinson's disease. Sugar causes the structure of collagen to change making skin age faster. Sugar has been connected with cancer of the breast, ovaries, prostate, rectum, pancreas, biliary tract, lung, gallbladder and stomach. Sugar can cause food allergies, eczema, and increase blood pressure. Sugar can decrease insulin sensitivity resulting in abnormally high insulin levels and eventually diabetes.

When sugar is heated with protein and fats as with most baked products, it produces harmful compounds called advanced glaciation end products. These can contribute to blood vessel damage, among other things. Some of us were born with a tendency towards certain diseases such as heart disease, certain cancers, diabetes, circulatory diseases, high blood pressure, stroke, and addictions from alcohol, to smoking, to food. These factors can cause you to either overproduce insulin or develop a resistance to it. Most people have both problems, overproduction followed by resistance on the cell receptors. Insulin is important to life and we must have it to live. However, if the pancreas wears out from the over-production because of the ineffectiveness of the resistant cell receptors, then what started out as a tendency towards hyperglycemia has moved into reactive hypoglycemia, and is on it's way to adult diabetes.

The term "adult diabetes" doesn't just apply to adults, because we are now seeing children diagnosed with this killer disease at early ages. Ninety-nine and-a-half percent of all women are addicted to sugar and most have a history of miserable bouts with PMS. One of the important hormones in the body is insulin, and when it is not working properly, the rest of your hormones don't work right either. The hyper-insulin problem is closely tied to female hormones.

The body has a very good memory system and can immediately re member what you ate and drank last year. This may be one of the reasons why sugar seems to have a more adverse affect on women than men, also making it harder for women to break the addiction. When the mineral balance in your body has been restored through the use of Celtic Salt, you will no longer have a craving for sugar or want sugary foods.

Milk and Dairy

Like everyone else, I grew up drinking more milk than water. In fact, I thought I needed milk every day, and felt bad if I didn't have it. With all of the commercials regarding milk and its healthy benefits, I was psyched into believing the hype. I didn't like milk, yet continued drinking it because I thought one needed it be healthy Despite having excess phlegm, mucus, and colds all the time, I was brainwashed by the dairy industry and their "gotta have milk" and calcium adds. When in fact, the incidence of calcium deficiencies is very rare in America, and is normally found in poor third-world countries. Over consumption of calcium from dairy products in particular has been linked to kidney stones, and cancer of the liver and colon. There is much talk about putting warning labels on milk, because it is no longer considered such a totally healthy substance. Dairy products are a health hazard to the overall human body be-cause they contain no fiber or complex carbohydrates, and are laden with saturated fat and cholesterol. They are contaminated with cow's blood and pus, and are frequently contaminated with pesticides, hor-mones, and antibiotics.

We, as humans, were not designed to drink the milk of other animals, yet humans are the only species who deliberately drink the milk of other animals. Domesticated pets will drink milk, but that is because they are taught to. Calves are taken from their mothers and fed formula, so that humans can have an adequate supply of milk in their diets. Cows are also impregnated and given dangerous growth hormones like Bovine, which enables them to produce milk continu-ously, greatly increasing dairy industry profits. Through genetic manipulation, most cows can produce a staggering 18,000 pounds of milk a year. That's more than three times their normal yearly pro-duction. Cows have a normal life span of 25 years, but are normally taken to slaughter in just five years because of the stress from over milking. The hormones adversely affect the health of the cows causing many birth defects, and may also cause breast and prostate cancer in humans, which has led to many countries banning its use. Dairy products are linked to allergies, constipation, obesity, heart disease, cancer, and other diseases. In addition to all the chemicals, antibiotics, growth hormones, and bacteria in milk, milk also coats your stomach and intestinal walls with a mucus-type film that, over time, thickens and turns into a plastic, rubbery-type substance.

If only I knew about the dangers of drinking milk. Fortunately I stopped drinking milk around the age of nine. I don't know why, but I just didn't feel comfortable drinking milk anymore. I replaced the milk in my cereal with fruit juices, and believe it or not, it tasted very good. You see, humans only need milk up until the age of three-and-a half to four. Because humans are premature compared to most other animals, we need milk after birth to finish our development outside the womb. Through nature, this process is completed with milk after birth. During the nine months we're in the womb, we feed on the nutrients found in milk. The milk we drink is just a continuation of this feeding to speed up development. Because we are beings of higher intelligence, we require larger brains, which require larger heads. If all humans were born fully developed, our heads wouldn't fit through the birth canal.

Milk forces premature cells of newly born infants to reproduce at very high rates of speed. For example at birth, an infant's heart only weighs about one ounce, compared to an adult heart weighing in at 500 ounces. It also beats twice as fast as a heart of an adult. All of this growing and activity requires a lot of energy to burn, and this energy is supplied by the mother's breast milk. At around two and-a-half to four years of age, the body automatically stops producing rennin, the enzyme secreted in the stomach to dissolve the protein casein from calcium so calcium can be absorbed into the body However, the calcium in pasturized milk is totally unusable by the body, causing the body to leach calcium from itself to neutralize the harmful amount of protein milk contains. Dr. Benjamin Spock, a leading authority on developing child health care, spoke against feeding cow's milk to children, saying it causes anemia, asthma, allergies, and insulin-dependent diabetes, and over time, can set children up for obesity and heart disease, the number one killer in America. Instead of preventing osteoporosis, it may cause this disease.

American women often consume very large amounts of calcium daily, yet their rates of osteoporosis are among the highest in the world. Conversely, Chinese women, consuming half the calcium(mostly from plant sources), have had scarce incidents of the bone disease. A Harvard Nurses' Study of more than 77,000 women found that those who consumed two or more glasses of milk per day had a higher risk of broken hips and arms than those who had one glass or less per day. A nutritional biochemistry professor at Cornell University stated that the link between the intake of animal protein and fracture rates appear to be as strong as that between cigarette smoking and lung cancer. Milk consumption is attributed to all of the following: diarrhea, heart disease, colic, cramps, gastrointestinal bleeding, sinusitis, diabetes, arthritis, acne, ear infections, osteoporosis, asthma, autoimmune disease and possibly lung cancer, multiple sclerosis, and non-Hodgkins lymphoma.

U.S. schools are required by law to put milk on every meal tray. All of the nutrients gotten from milk can be had from other foods like plants, raw almonds, nuts, fruits, legumes, seeds, yeast, tofu, and regular sunshine. Because the body can't use milk, it will sit in the stomach undigested. It then passes over into the colon where bacteria ferment it, converting it into gas and lactate acid (milk sugars). When the body doesn't have enough energy to eliminate this dairy product, it stores it in the joints and we call it arthritis. If we store it in the liver, we call it cirrhosis. If it is stored as a clump, it is called a tumor. What do we call big chunks of protein and calcium stuck in your kidney? Kidney stones. What does your doctor tell you to stop consuming if you suffer with kidney stones? Milk and dairy. Why don't we simply stop eating dairy products so we don't get kidney stones to begin with?

Women who reported consuming skim or low-fat milk every day had a 66% higher risk of developing ovarian cancer. The near-vegetarian women of Papua, New Guinea, drink no milk after weaning, and have the lowest incidence of osteoporosis in the world. Dairy products go through a process called homogenization, which scars the arteries in your body. Is it no wonder then that heart disease is the number one killer in North America, Canada, and Europe. Like I said before, it doesn't take a brain scientist or a Ph.D. There are many other things you can drink to replace milk, like almond, soy, and rice beverages. Again, in my opinion, we should look to nature and follow her wisdom, and put processed milk aside for healthier choices.

Commercially Processed Bread and Wheat Products

Bread, in biblical days, was considered the staff of life. Today, you can accurately term bread made from white flour the taker of life, contributing to wide-spread vitamin and mineral deficiencies. The three major ingredients of modern bread are white flour, sugar, and hydrogenated oils. All of the more than 30 naturally occurring vitamins, minerals, and nutrients are removed, and a lot of bad stuff is added, then we wonder why everyone in this country is sick. One slice of white bread has 65% less fiber, magnesium and potassium than whole-wheat bread. The bran alone in whole-wheat bread gives it 20 times more antioxidant power than a diet high in refined grains, which carry a higher risk of stroke, weight gain, Type II diabetes and heart disease. A diet high in whole grains has been linked to lower incidents of heart disease, weight gain, Type II diabetes, and colon cancer. Whole grains also appear to increase insulin sensitivity used to balance blood sugar levels. On the flip side, refined grains seem to cause unhealthy spikes in blood which can lead to Type II diabetes

Today, more than three-fourths of the dietary fiber is removed from commercial flour resulting in more frequent cases of constipation. Vital nutrients which are removed and not returned include vitamin E, pantothenic and folic acid, biotin, vitamin B_6, and 20 minerals and trace mineral elements, including all magnesium, calcium, zinc, chromium, manganese, selenium, vanadium, zinc, and copper. A chemical similar to Clorox bleach is also added to help turn this worthless mess white at the expense of your health. This bleaching process leaves behind traces of toxic residue that causes nervousness and seizures in animals. The bleaching process destroys any remaining nutrients that might be left. Germany has banned the bleaching of bread since 1958.

Ninety-five percent of all white flour used in bread, rolls, cakes, pastries, spaghetti, noodles, pasta, and breakfast cereals, have been bleached. To extend needed shelf life, chemicals are added like ethylated mono and triglycerides, potassium bromate, potassium iodide, calcium propionate, benzoyl peroxide, tricalcium phosphate, calcium sulfate, ammonium chloride and magnesium carbonate. The only mineral put back in bread is iron, which research has shown can cause all kinds of health conditions like atherosclerosis, heart attacks, strokes and arthritis. Various medical writers on food allergies and allergic poisoning say that wheat is the most common food to which patients have shown sensitivity. Diseases and conditions that can be caused by eating bread and other processed wheat products are altered liver function, anemia, cancer, difficulty breathing, heart disease, impaired vision, multiple sclerosis, obesity, polio, rheumatic fever, and rheumatoid arthritis.

Coffee

Coffee lovers, grin and weep. I don't want to ruin your party, but the caffeine in coffee is actually a an anti-fungal agent. It acts as a pesticide assumed to be part of the plant's defense mechanism to keep away insects. When it gets into your system, it revs you up and makes you feel good right? What's actually happening is it's speeding up your metabolism to process the poisons out quicker, and drawing water out of the body to first dilute the poison and then eliminate as a diuretic. This process uses up energy and hastens the aging process. Drinking decaf is no different than regular coffee.

Water

Water is something we all take for granted. We are told to drink spring water and fluoridated water; however, our bodies were designed and work best when we drink purified or distilled water. The only difference between the two is that purified water has minerals added back into it, distilled doesn't. The minerals added back are not in their natural state, so the best water to drink is distilled water. If you want the extra benefit of the minerals, simply add a few of shakes of Celtic Sea Salt to your water before drinking it. Some spring water contains parasites unless it has been treated through the process of reverse osmosis, which is probably how the majority of the water you buy in grocery stores is processed. Ninety-seven percent of the water on this earth is locked away in the oceans and is undrinkable, making it toxic to humans, animals, and some plants. The sun heats up waters in our rivers, lakes, and oceans, turning it into purified water vapor which rises into the air. When the water vapor cools, it forms clouds, which become heavy with water and rain back to the earth. This purified water then washes and cleanses the earth. In this same manner, we need purified water to wash toxins away that build up in our bodies, blood, and cells.

Soda

Soda or "liquid candy" as it should be called contains as much as 16 teaspoons of sugar per can. Just one teaspoon of sugar will shut down your immune system for up to twelve hours. The majority of us go the whole week without using our immune systems. Is it any wonder then why so many people suffer with colds in this country. Soda has been linked to obesity, tooth decay, weakened bones, and caffeine addictions. Soda sales account for 1/4 of all drinks sold in the United States, more than 15 billion gallons annually. Studies indicate that diets high in sugary foods like soft drinks may increase the risk of heart disease in insulin-resistant adults. Other research has linked soda consumption to kidney stones in men. Soft drink companies have spent over $6 billion in the past decade just on advertising. They pay big bucks for exclusive marketing rights to schools. Coca-Cola was paying the Boys & Girls Club of America some $60 million to make its products the only brand sold in more than 2,000 clubs. Diet drinks are more worrisome due to artificial sweeteners like saccharin that may promote cancer. The average American spends $54 billion a year on pop. That's twice the amount spent on books in this country.

Smoking

In a recent Surgeon General's report, it stated that smoking is attributed to acute myeloid leukemia and cancers of the cervix, kidney, pancreas, stomach, abdominal aneurysm, cataracts, pneumonia, and chronic bronchitis. Smokers die an average of 13 to 14 years earlier than non-smokers. Prior diseases linked to smoking are cancer of the bladder, esophagus, larynx, lungs, mouth, and throat. Smoking has also been linked to chronic lung disease as well as reproductive problems. About 440,000 Americans die of smoking-related diseases each year, and some 12 million people have died in the past 40 years. The cost of treating smoking-related diseases and loss of productivity is a staggering $160 billion annually. In a recent study, medical researchers collecting data in the state of Colorado reported a 27% drop in deaths due to heart attacks in areas of the state that were zoned as smoke free.

Artificial Sweeteners

All artificial sweeteners are chemical drugs that are labeled as food, which is a major problem. Because they're considered a food and consumed in massive amounts that the body can't throw off, these sweeteners interfere with all hormonal and chemical processes that naturally occur in the body. The greatest concern anyone should have eating foods containing this unhealthy product are the unknown long-term affects they can have on the body.

As I mentioned earlier, saccharin was touted as being safe even though it was proven to cause bladder cancer in laboratory rats. It has been mostly removed from the food supply, but the point still remains, these chemicals are dangerous to humans. If it's man made and stripped of all nutritional value, don't eat it. Use all natural sweeteners that are easily assimilated in the body like stevia, maple syrup and honey.

Washing Your Hands

This habit is the easiest and most effective way to avoid the spread of unhealthy bacteria. Most bacteria and viruses cannot live outside of a living host. For example, the AIDS virus will quickly die if exposed to air. What amazes me is the fact that so many believers today come out of church, shake hands with everybody, and then nonchalantly eat and put things in their mouths without a thought of washing their hands. All believers should wash their hands as they exit the church and especially before sitting down to eat. In the Bible, there are countless references in the Old and New Testaments regarding the washing of hands and feet.

Fluoride

The two most common sources of fluoride in this country are toothpaste and fluoridated water. Fluoride is not biodegradable so it accumulates in the body and bones, resulting in toxic poisoning. This is why toothpaste containing fluoride comes with the following required warning "WARNINGS: Keep out of reach of children under 6 years of age. If you accidentally swallow more than is used for brushing, seek professional help or contact the Poison Control Center immediately." Just a half of tube of toothpaste can cause the accidental death of a child and cause severe demineralization of both bone and tooth enamel in adults. A 1970 study found a high incident in bone structure defects in Newburgh, N.Y., one of the first communities in the country to fluoridate its water. Fluoride is actually a toxic drug not made for human consumption, in some cases causing heart and muscle problems. This is what happens when mankind tries to tamper with what God has created naturally. Fluoride that is naturally occurring in Celtic Sea Salt is in very minute quantities and is balanced by the more than 80 other minerals and trace minerals.

Plan Your Meals

Plan your meals in advance so that you don't just buy whatever you see as you do your shopping. Preplan up to 15 of your favorite dishes which can be prepared in 30 minutes or less. Shop the outside aisles of the supermarket first where most of the healthier foods are located. This will also ensure upon reaching your spending limit, you'll have more healthy items in the basket than unhealthy junk foods. Avoid pre-packaged frozen dinners such as diet meals, T.V. dinners, cakes and pies. These meals may appear to be healthy, but they are actually loaded with many artificial preservatives, chemical additives, sodium, and artificial sweeteners that may not be listed. They also contain deadly trans fats or partially hydrogenated oils.

Trans fats have already been linked to heart disease, obesity, cancer and diabetes to name a few. It's amazing the number of frozen healthy dinners that are available, yet the number of people diagnosed with degenerative diseases is continuing to rise. These meals will never be able to replace the awesome health benefits that one can receive from eating whole raw unprocessed foods. It is best to prepare your own meals and only eat frozen meals as a last resort. Avoid canned goods because they contain virtually no nutritional value, and are loaded with sodium and artificial sweeteners. Fresh is always best, and has the greatest benefits overall. **Remember, God has placed before you life and death, sickness and disease, so choose life, that you and your seed may live.**

CHAPTER 12

How do I Save Myself and My Family

"I have set before you life and death, blessing and cursing: therefore choose life, that both thou and thy seed may live:" (Deuteronomy 30:19)

In the 12th chapter of Genesis, we are introduced to the father of faith, Abraham. Here we meet him long before he receives his new name from God. At this point, his name is Abram, meaning exalted father. He doesn't know that one day he will be the father of many multitudes. In order for God to prepare him for this change, Abram had to be removed, relocated, and transformed out of his environment, and into a land that God would show him. Genesis 12:1 says, "Now the Lord had said unto Abram, get thee out of thy country, and from the kindred, and from thy father's house, unto a land I will show thee." Abram's lifestyle and historical influences were not conducive to God's plan for his life. So he had to be physically transplanted and mentally transformed. He had too much unhealthy history and influences surrounding him. Too many unhealthy generational traditions passed down to him from his ancestors. By allowing him to remain around his kindred, it would have given him the propensity to digress back into the same lifestyle that God wanted him to avoid.

Today, almost 4500 years later, many of us are just like Abraham. We are influenced by historical traditions that are not conducive to God's plan for our lives. Now because we haven't transformed our minds, the condition of our health continues to deteriorate. We have conformed to the ways of the world, so we have many questions, but no answers. We continue down the same path that has taken the lives of so many of our loved ones. As is the case involving the half-ton man, whose father and grandfather weighed a combined 600 pounds. His ancestors' unhealthy lifestyle choices eventually became a part of his environment, greatly impacting his life to the point of bringing him just weeks away from certain death. Yes, this man's historical generational habits caused him to eat himself to death.

Although he may not have died physically, living in his condition wasn't really living at all. If he was going to save himself, he should have realized he needed to be relocated, and transform his thoughts and perceptions regarding certain types of food.

What's frightening is the fact that today, many of us have classified certain diseases and then tied them to our lives. "Oh, cancer runs in their family," or "heart disease is on my side of the family." In Abraham's family, it was the fact that his ancestors worshiped idol gods, which spiritually is just as deadly as cancer or heart disease. Despite this spiritual disease on his side of the family, there was still hope for him and his condition was not terminal. This story speaks volumes to us today, because just like Abraham, our condition is not terminal just as long as we are willing to transform ourselves out of our familiar traditions and habits; if we are willing to do some self examining, and put aside practices or gods that compromise our health.

There are five common denominators that seem to be connected to every major sickness, illness, disease, and chronic affliction. It seems that if these five elements are present in any community, undue suffering and sickness will be present also. There will be more incidents of cancer, diabetes, arthritis, heart disease, osteoporosis, eczema, Alzheimer's disease, fibromyalgia, high cholesterol, muscle cramps, kidney stones and failure, gallstones, gout, indigestion, chronic fatigue syndrome, weight problems, lupus, acne, acid reflux, circulation disorders, hypertension, heartburn, high blood pressure, violence, muscular dystrophy, learning disorders, obesity, and a whole host of other diseases. The five common culprits are refined sugar, dehydration or lack of water, mineral-deficient table salt, trans fats, and lack of exercise. People who live in areas where these five elements are prevalent seem to always suffer from some type of physical or psychological illness. I believe these five common denominators are responsible for up to 80% of all undue afflictions in this country, and in other countries that are starting to follow our western dietary lifestyle. As the nutritional habits here in the west start to take hold abroad, more and more countries are starting to see a dramatic rise in the number of chronic illnesses.

This is evidenced by the fact that women living in Japan, China and Asia have very low incidence of breast cancer. However, when they move to America and start eating western foods, their chances of developing breast cancer is just the same as American women. This study was later confirmed when scientists discovered that Japanese men who moved to Hawaii had increased incidents of cancer upon adding American processed foods to their diets. When commercially processed American foods, which are full of refined salt, arrived in Africa, soon afterward something hardly ever seen before arrived with it, cancer. In all three cases, the only thing that really changed was the condition of the food. The people didn't go through any type of metaphysical changes. They simply were exposed to processed and mineral depleted foods.

Because all nutrients are dependent upon minerals to function and interact with each other, an absence of minerals can cause major problems. These nationalities transformed their way of life as it relates to location and nutrition, and all had the same results and increased rate of certain types of cancers. If people could somehow manage these areas, chronic illnesses would start disappearing around the world. People would live longer and healthier lives, with a greater state of mental and emotional stability. I want us to journey into these five areas and dissect how each plays a major contributing factor, and the domino affects they cause. You will see that diabetes, obesity, cancer, heart disease, hypertension, and kidney failure, are all connected with these five common denominators. The first is a white, crystallized substance that is found in just about 95% of all processed foods. It is an unnatural substance found nowhere in nature and causes more health problems than any other food or drug in the world. As more and more cultures around the globe incorporate these white crystals into their normal diets, they are starting to deal with illnesses never before seen in their countries. As I said earlier, diabetes and obesity affect some 300 million people around the world. This mysterious substance is called white sugar, and is so alien, the human body doesn't even recognize it as a nutritional substance it can use. It is completely stripped of all nutrients, then bleached white and sold as food. This white poison is highly addictive and habit forming, just like another deadly drug called heroin.

As I am writing this book, roughly 95% of this country's population is addicted to sugar and crave it all the time. Sugar's slow and insidious damage has caused more harm than all natural disasters to hit this country combined. Last year, the cost to treat sugar-related illnesses was $400 billions, and those who didn't die are still suffering.

its affects. Sugar is a major contributor to diabetes, obesity, hypertension, cardiovascular disease, cancer, compromised immune ability, weakened bones, elevated cholesterol levels, poor vision, poor teeth, uncontrolled growth of candida yeast, and over 130 other illnesses.

One problem with sugar is that once it enters the body, it turns highly acidic which causes the whole body to deprive itself of oxygen. Human life is built on the need for oxygen. When it is lacking, degenerative sickness, disease and eventually death will result. Sugar in very small quantities wouldn't harm us much, especially if we drank more water. Instead, we eat large amounts of sugar or refined food products, which are also loaded with sugar. In both cases, through industrial processing, all of the vital nutrients are removed from foods to prevent spoilage. After the food is stripped of nutrients and fiber, refined sugar is added to preserve it. If you pour sugar into your gas tank, it will kill your engine. Now imagine what it will do in your body. The first major problem we have is the fact that our bodies are overexposed to too much sugar, which is highly acidic. Keeping our bodies exposed to this condition for an extended period of time is very unhealthy.

The next is dehydration or lack of water, which should probably be at the top of the list. Some people are under the impression that by drinking soda, coffee, espresso, milk shakes, and fruit juices all day that they are actually satisfying their need for water, which is one of the reasons why so many of us are suffering with failing health issues. For some reason, no one feels the need to drink clean, refreshing water. Water is so vitally important to our survival that God turned bitter water into sweet drinkable water in Exodus 15:25. He also welled water from rocks as the Israelites wandered for 40 years in the wilderness. Now God had just parted the Red Sea, so He could have miraculously fulfilled their physical need for water without actually giving them water to drink. However that would void the validity and integrity of His word. God created us from water and He created water for us. The body is comprised of almost 75% water. Isn't it amazing how well the body responds to water, and will even signal you when dehydration starts to set in. Water regulates body temperature and is a natural insulator. A person can live for more than a month without food, but only one week without water. Water flushes and cleanses your cells and blood of waste materials, toxins, etc. It then flushes this waste out through the kidneys and bowels. We will wash our clothes and cars with water, but won't wash out our cells. Your cells deserve better treatment than your clothes for without living cells, you won't need clothes to wear or a car to drive.

Nothing can take the place of fresh, clean water. Every living organism on earth must have water in some form in order to survive. The brain is composed of 70% water, while the lungs are up to 90% water. Our blood is 85% water and the average person must replace 2.5 liters of water daily. People who are physically active can lose up to 10 liters of water per day. Water is unique in that it has the ability to dissolve so many substances. More than 20,000 healthy men and women were studied by researchers at Loma Linda University in Southern California. They found that those who drank more than five glasses of water a day were less likely to die from heart attack or heart disease than those who drank fewer than two glasses a day.

Here are a few more reasons why we all should drink more water. Water moisturizes your skin, is essential to maintaining elasticity and suppleness, and helps prevent dryness. Water can help you control weight by preventing you from confusing hunger with thirst. It will keep your metabolism and digestion working properly and give you energy. By helping to flush toxins, appropriate water intake lessens the burden on your kidneys and liver, lubricates and cushions your joints and muscles. Water helps prevent constipation by adding fluid to the colon and bulk to stools. It has the remarkable ability of helping to prevent headaches and improves concentration. Water can help prevent kidney stones and reduce your chances of getting infections. One study found that women who drank more than five glasses of water a day had a risk of colon cancer that was 45% less than those who drank two or fewer glasses a day. Water can help control fevers, replace lost fluids, and thin out mucus.

The third and deadliest culprit, which ranks right next to dehydration, is the consumption of mineral-depleted salts. The condition of our salt today is actually a health hazard in and of itself. It is absolutely dangerous to your health and should be avoided at all costs. More than sugar, this is probably the most serious health risk facing many countries in the world. The refinement of our salt here in America actually causes our bodies to leach minerals when it should be supplying us with vitally needed minerals. Yes, we are supposed to get a fresh supply of minerals everyday, just like water, to replace the ones that are constantly being lost. Losing minerals is not such a bad thing as long as they are replaced. Our problem to day is we don't ever replace the ones that are being lost, and the food we eat leaches and destroys whatever minerals we have remaining in our bodies.

We are also faced with the medical community telling us to avoid salt altogether, especially minorities with high blood pressure. This advice, while helping to control blood pressure, now leads to kidney failure. Without natural sea salt, the kidneys have to work harder to keep the body flushed. This overburdening of the kidneys, along with an acidic diet, weakens and debilitates them over time. In all actuality, it is not the salt that is causing the problems, but the condition of the salt. Humans can't remain healthy for very long without salt, because we need the minerals in real sea salt for all of our bodily functions. After salt has been refined, only two minerals remain. Then it is mixed with other highly toxic substances and heavy metals. We poison ourselves as we consume excessive amounts through our food supply. We have nothing in our diets to counter the affects of the salt. So it builds up in the cells and tissues of our bodies. Some of it is stored as cellulite, especially in people who live a sedentary lifestyle. Refined table salt defiles and poisons the blood, and causes all kinds of physical and mental manifestations.

There are severe mineral deficiencies of magnesium, selenium, and lithium in this country today. Magnesium is one of the main components of all living matter. It stimulates white blood cell activity and promotes the action of vitamins, just to name a few of its vital functions in the body. Magnesium scarcity is the cause of many diseases. All junk foods and refined white products like white bread and refined grain products are magnesium deficient. Selenium is another very important mineral antioxidant. Its deficiency has been linked to higher levels of heart disease, cancer, AIDS, and even miscarriages. Humans, along with animals, have been exposed to viruses and bacteria since the creation of mankind. The green monkeys and two other species of monkeys, considered to be the origin of HIV, are heavily infected with SIV, the original of HIV. Yet they are all immune to the disease. This proves indisputably that an effective immune system can deal with viruses and overcome them. Humans have caught and consumed animal flesh and so to have been exposed to the SIV virus for thousands of years. In essence, we should be just as immune to SIV and HIV as the green monkeys.

As I stated earlier, the only thing that has changed in recent history or within the last few decades is the defilement and depletion of minerals from our soils and food supply. It might well be the culmination of decades of selenium depletion and deficiency, including a daily diet of immune suppressing refined foods like white flour, table salt, refined sugar, rice, pasta, soda, etc., instead of consuming whole and all natural unbleached mineral-rich foods. Although the green monkeys are immune to SIV in the wild, they come down with SIV shortly after being captured and brought into our laboratories and fed our severely-trace elements and selenium-deficient foods.

The third is lithium, a trace mineral properly balanced in Celtic Sea Salt. Psychiatrists use lithium in two ways: to treat episodes of mania and depression and to prevent their recurrence. Lithium can often subdue symptoms when a patient is in the midst of a manic episode, and it may also ameliorate the symptoms of a depressive episode. The single most important use for lithium, though, is in preventing new episodes of mania and depression. Lithium is highly effective in treating acute episodes of mania, especially when symptoms are mild. Patients going through severe manic episodes need to be calmed as quickly as possible, however, and lithium may take one to three weeks to achieve its full effect. Lithium can normalize the manic disorder without causing the drugged feeling that often occurs with tranquilizers. Lithium is also effective in treating depressive episodes in some patients with manic-depressive illness. As noted, lithium's greatest value is in preventing or reducing the occurrences of future episodes of bipolar disorder. The effectiveness of this lithium treatment has been demonstrated in more than two decades of careful research. In related research, several major studies indicate that lithium can decrease the frequency or severity of new depressive episodes in recurrent unipolar disorder.

These are just three of the more than 85 minerals that are currently missing from our food supply. You don't have to have a Ph.D. to connect the dots here. Both refined salt and sugar are linked to causing the same type of degenerative diseases. Since their introduction into the food supply, degenerative diseases and mental disorders have increased proportionately with increased usage of both substances. It appears that as more and more minerals are removed orders have increased proportionately with increased usage of both substances. It appears that as more and more minerals are removed from the food supply, the incidents of mental and physical disorders are steadily rising. The bigger picture here is that we are consuming mineral-deficient foods that are also mineral depleting. In this condition, we are really just empty vessels of clay, and although we may look beautiful on the outside, there is nothing working on the inside. It wouldn't be so bad except for the fact that we don't drink enough water either. I won't go into too much detail regarding the fourth culprit which, in my opinion, is the deadliest synthetic substance ever created-"trans fats" or hydrogenated oils. I have covered this one extensively in **Chapter 5.** However, just the last three culprits alone should sound the alarm.

Now we will briefly examine culprit number five, which is also extensively covered in **Chapter 13.** Lack of exercise and physical activity have caused the healthcare costs in this country to spiral out of control. Everyone is affected, because in one way or another, we are paying to treat this condition everyday. That's right. You may work out two hours a day and be as strong as an ox. However, you still are not exempt, because you are footing the bill for the laziness of someone else. In my opinion, we all should exercise daily as this will ensure the constant removal of excess waste and toxins from the blood.

Remember, the life of the flesh is in the blood. It is a verifiable fact that people who exercise (all age groups) suffer with less sicknesses of every type than those who do not. Exercise improves the overall condition of the entire body, both internally and externally. There are three things that God made sure the Israelites were exposed to while wandering through the desert. They had water, a salty environment, and plenty of exercise. They had to gather and prepare manna everyday for 40 years. If these three elements were important for them, then they're certainly essential to us.

So there you have it, the five most dangerous things that we can all change starting right now to save our health and that of our precious loved ones. I know you probably thought it was going to be something very deep and complicated. Now the real truth of the matter is it's really just that simple. If you don't believe me, I dare you to try it for just 30 days and see if you don't feel better and more energetic than you've felt in years. In fact, it won't even take

30 days. You'll start feeling a difference immediately. Listen, for the past 10, 20, 40, 60, or more years, you've been destroying the temple. How about letting the temple have a well-deserved break and give back 30 days of your health to God. All degenerative diseases, including autoimmune diseases, can be reversed and healed. Listen, you must use wisdom and not your taste buds. The five major culprits I mentioned are just the beginning of a major step in the right direction. Properly correcting these imbalances will save you and your loved ones untold misery, suffering, and wealth. Take the savings you accumulate from healthier living and put it into a retirement account or a college savings plan for your children and grand-children.

As you start removing and transforming yourself as it relates to these five major culprits mentioned above, there are five healthy common counter denominators such as garlic, olive oil, Celtic Sea Salt, water, and seed extracts which you can cheaply and easily implement into your lifestyle that can help the body remain healthy and prevent disease. Garlic is one of the oldest medicinal herbs known to mankind, and for a change, it is mentioned in the Bible. Garlic has been used as both a food and medicine by cultures worldwide for more than 5,000 years. Garlic contains sulfur compounds, B vitamins, minerals, flavonoids, various amino acids, proteins, lipids, steroids, and 12 trace elements.

There are more than 880 remedies associated with the use of Garlic. Egyptian men working on the pyramids revolted because their daily rations of garlic were cut back. Garlic is beneficial for the entire body and is recommended to treat infections, wounds, leprosy, cancer, digestive disorders, coughs, clearing arteries, lowering blood pressure, treat dysentery, colds, parasites, poisoning, and improving overall cholesterol levels. One of the most powerful affects of garlic is its ability to greatly enhance the immune system. Raw, fresh, organic garlic should be taken every day or at least every other day continuously.

First cold press, extra virgin olive oil should be taken once a day. It contains very powerful medicinal properties and is effective in balancing the body's pH. Olive oil is also great for the entire body, especially the skin. Olive oil protects against certain types of cancer as well as other degenerative diseases. The raw fats of the olive oil lubricates cells, joints, intestines, and arteries. They help aid with digestion, making foods assimilate easier. There are hundreds of other benefits of olive oil that time will not permit me to cover. Celtic Sea Salt is covered extensively in **Chapter 11.** I can't say it enough. You absolutely need real mineral-balanced sea salt in your diet daily. If you don't have all-natural Celtic Sea Salt, you are doing yourself more harm than good. Jesus commands that we be salted and use salt until He returns. Sprinkle salt on all your foods and even into your water as you start drinking more of it. Remember, all salt is not the same. It must say 100% pure, unrefined, and tested Celtic Sea Salt. Without replenishing the body of its natural mineral reserves, you will greatly compromise your body's structural integrity and overall well being.

Water, water, water, and then some more water. Enough cannot be said about the need to drink at least six to eight glasses of pure distilled water every day. Put down the soda, milk, coffee, cappuccinos, commercial fruit juices, and pick up the water. With as many poisons and toxins that we allow to enter our bodies, we need all the water we can get our hands on. Water is great because it continuously flushes the internal oceans within the body and protects our cellular environments at the same time.

Last, but definitely not least, are seed extracts, in particular grape fruit and grapefruit seed. These are two of the most potent disease fighting nutrients on the planet. We may also add pomegranate seeds which are also very potent. Seed extracts produce wellness and healing for the entire body. They have been proven to stop and prevent certain cancers from developing altogether. They are also a part of our original diet according to Genesis 1:29. If they worked for the patriarchs, I'm certainly willing to give them a chance. What about you? Recently, Oprah Winfrey aired a special about heart disease being the number one killer of women in this country. Each moment that you are reading this book, someone's mother, sister, aunt, daughter, niece, or grandmother has died from heart disease. A woman dies of heart disease every minute for an annual total of about half a million per year.

I want to take this moment to challenge every artist, singer, rapper, and actor. These women who are dying or will die are the same women who are cast in your music videos and movies. The women we don't see are the millions of women watching and buying your products. The next time you shoot a movie, music video, or produce a CD, devote one track or clip to drop a word of knowledge to all our women, providing vital information about preventing and reversing heart disease. Believe me, It won't cut into your sales if you have one track that's devoted to the saving of a life. With all the scenes of women being used as sex objects, gyrating their bodies before the cameras, what better way to show your appreciation than to devote just one music track to show how much you really care. The women in your movie or music video is some little girl's mother or some mother's daughter. With your exposure and talents, you could be very affective in sounding the alarm, and help to start reversing this degenerative disease. If I can do my part with less than a 10th of a 10th of your resources. I'm quite sure you can pitch in just a little. If you asked every female fan out there about this idea, they would back it 100%. Who knows, it may even help boost your sales.

There is definitely a famine in the land and the results are all around us. In times past, just a couple of decades or so ago, if you wanted to see a group of sick people congregated together at any given time, you either had to take a visit to a hospital or local nursing home. What a big difference a few decades can make, because that is no longer the case. As you read this book, America is the wealthiest and sickest country on the planet. Instead of America the Beautiful, it should be called America the Medicated. More than half of all television commercials today are advertisements about some new drug with warnings of life-threatening complications caused by their side affects. Again, I cannot stress enough the fact that all medications are toxic and poisonous to the human body, especially the liver and kidneys. Satan has removed the minerals from our soils which affects all plants, animals, and humans. He has also removed it from the salt and from our bodies by giving us refined sugar, and other mineral leaching chemicals that are added to our food supply.

With that said, we all should stop blessing foods that don't bless us. We need to stop medicating ourselves with toxic drugs that give us a warning about more severe complications. If you read the warning label on a bottle of drain cleaner, you wouldn't think twice about not drinking it. All medications come with warning labels. You should apply the same caution to them as you do with drain cleaners. Celebrex, Plavix, Avandia, Vesicare- these drugs come with multiple side affects just to treat one disease. Sometimes the side affects are worse than the ailment you are being treated for.

We must do all that we can to keep the integrity of our three internal oceans– blood plasma, lymphatic fluid, and extracellular fluid clean and balanced at all times as this will keep the rest of the body healthy and vibrant. Hydration and circulation are very important since all cells throw off waste that must be circulated out of the body. Gastric bypass surgery is not the answer, because it doesn't help the lymphatic system in removing waste from the blood. Without removing waste from the blood, arteries become clogged leading to heart disease. A recent report revealed that African American patients in particular, and other minorities who suffer heart attacks, have much higher rates of mortality upon being admitted to hospitals. With a new degenerative artery disease popping up every time you turn around, the last thing you want to worry about is dying from a heart attack just because you are a minority.

I wonder how Moses would react if he could see the horrible condition that our health has deteriorated into. Remember, the Bible states the he had full vigor and sight at the age of 120. I really can't imagine Christ returning to a sick, dying, and totally defeated body of sick believers. Every year, there is an outbreak of anthrax on the uninhabited planes of Africa, and after killing thousand of wildebeests, the seasonal rains come through and wash it all away. It doesn't make news here because no humans are affected by it. The point I am making here is that there is nothing that God has not already prepared the earth for. No new viruses, bacteria, or infectious diseases can totally wipe mankind from the face of the earth. So don't follow all the hype. Be truly led by the Spirit in all things.

If anyone has taken notice, you no longer have to visit a hospital or nursing home to see sick and dying people. Simply open your front door and step outside for a breath of fresh air, and you'll overhear someone's story about how their health is starting or has started to deteriorate. Or visit your local grocery store, mall, or Wal-Mart and you will be surrounded by sick looking and dying people driving or pushing shopping carts full of the foods that have helped facilitate their illnesses. They're dragging themselves round, operating motorized vehicles as they traverse the aisles attached to oxygen machines. If you don't see any of these images, somewhere in their purses, pockets, or on their possession you'll find all types of prescription medications. People carry around medicine today just as much as they carry money.

As a matter of fact, some people will walk around without a dime in their pockets, but will have their supply of medications handy. These people are not struck by lightening nor were they hit by a speeding freight train. They aren't born with polio or scarlet fever. I mean if this were the case, it would all make a lot of sense and I wouldn't be publishing this book. Now just the opposite is happening, which is destroying the very fabric of this country, forcing American companies to seek healthier employees overseas to remain competitive and profitable.

The record number of people currently suffering and dying are not the result of a natural disaster. These people were not being struck by lightening, hit by freight trains, or born with infectious diseases. They are suffering as a direct result of what they eat, drink, smoke, breathe, and bathe in. They are eating and drinking things that do not give them life, but actually destroys their lives and their loved ones. What really upsets me is the same conglomerates that processed the foods to make us sick now want to all of a sudden skip out and send jobs overseas. Due to the staggering rise in healthcare costs, it's inconveniently costing too much in corporate profits, so now they want to layoff employees, reduce pay, cut pension allotments, and leave us out to dry. That's right. For years, our food supply has been poisoned, all in the name of corporate profits.

Today, tap water from your kitchen sink is so unsafe that water treatment plants are scrambling to find chemical cleansers strong enough to remove toxic residue from the water. Trace amounts of certain medications are not being broken down in the water during treatment, because conventional cleansers aren't strong enough to dissolve them. As a result, these residues are recycled right back to your homes. The awful smelling stench being emitted from our water treatment plants today should be all you need as a signal. If you haven't stopped drinking tap water yet, don't drink another drop ever again unless you absolutely must.

These conglomerates who are contaminating the food supply are some of the same companies that lied about nicotine-addicting cigarettes. Chemicals were deliberately added to tobacco to make it more desirable and harder to kick. The evidence was secretly hidden behind the doors of corporate boardrooms. Now there are billions of dollars in lawsuits pending around the country. Yes, these corporations have gotten richer and we have gotten sicker. As if that weren't enough, these conglomerates are cutting back on pensions, paychecks, and jobs due to fact that healthcare costs have become a liability, and production has been lost due to the record number of sick employees. These industrial culprits want to now turn their backs on the American work force and their families. The same companies who have become extremely wealthy at the expense of our health now want to abandon us by taking our jobs, and sending them to countries overseas where the general population is not sick and dying; a place where the skyrocketing rise in healthcare costs will not eat into their bottom line, their corporate profits.

We haven't changed in our physical makeup since the creation of mankind. Our hearts, liver, kidneys, lungs, and the rest of our inner terrain has remained pretty much the same. We still breathe in air through our nostrils and blink our eyelids to retain moisture just like our ancestors. Even our outer environment has remained relatively unchanged since the creation of mankind. The trees still take in carbon dioxide and give us oxygen. We still eat from the same type of trees that fed Adam and Eve in the Garden of Eden. Humans will yet die of dehydration without water as has been the case since creation. The sun still provides light and warms the earth, the rain still falls from the clouds. So everything as it relates to creation is pretty much the same. The same type of grapes that Noah used to make wine are grown in vineyards all around the world today. Our ancestors used fire to heat their caves and cook foods in the same way that we use fire today to heat our homes and cook also. So if nothing has really changed physically or environmentally, then what is causing the historical levels of chronic diseases now facing mankind.

It appears that almost every week, there is a television commercial describing some newly discovered disease with a medical treatment to go along with it. It is scary to think that 24 hours a day, we are bombarded with commercials advocating the use of drugs to treat every ailment. Prayer is not ever mentioned as an alternative treatment, even though it causes no adverse side affects. This country has been shaped by television for decades, influencing everything from the clothes we wear to the smoking of cigarettes, from super-sized meals to the explosion of sexual promiscuity propagated by

Hollywood. Just let television promote it, and the rest of the population will soon follow suit, including some believers.

Today, it appears as though television is being used to promote the use of medication as the answer to all the ills of mankind. Got a problem, just pop a pill and go about your business. In the not too distant future, we will all be shaped into legalized drug addicts, monopolized by those who run the pharmaceutical conglomerates. If nothing has changed, then why are so many people suffering from degenerative diseases? Scripture attests to the fact that mankind was able to live in a sinful state for decades and still enjoy good health and longevity. If we haven't changed physically, then we must look deeper into what we allow to enter our bodies. The one thing that has changed since creation is the condition of our soils, which has negatively impacted the nutritional value of our foods.

Yes, to sum it all up, the food we eat and the way it is processed has dramatically changed over the past 100 years. Added to this is the fact that we are not physically active, and we don't drink enough water. So again, it all goes right back to the choices we make. If these choices are the cause of our problems, then we can reverse these same choices and heal ourselves with an all-natural approach. This approach will be a lot less taxing on your body, bank accounts, and your loved ones. This approach will also help you recover while suffering fewer side affects. **Remember, God has placed before you life and death, sickness and disease, so choose life, that you and your seed may live.**

Exercise! Exercise! Exercise!

"I have set before you life and death, blessing and cursing: therefore choose life, that both thou and thy seed may live:" (Deuteronomy 30:19)

- Over 150 million people are overweight.

- Over 14 million people have adult-onset Type II diabetes.

- Over 150,000 people are diagnosed with colon cancer per year.

- Over 16 million people have coronary heart disease.

- Over 2 million people suffer from a heart attack in a given year, with 499,000 women actually dying.

- Over 300,000 people suffer from hip fractures each year.

- Over 70 million people have high blood pressure.

Jesus walked 90 miles to a wedding where He performed His first miracle, turning water into wine. He also hiked over 9,000 feet to the peak of a summit, and upon reaching the summit, Jesus was transfigured, and worshiped His heavenly father along with Moses, Elijah, and three of His disciples. Jonah had to walk over 90 miles to reach Nineveh after being delivered from the belly of a whale. Believe it or not, back in biblical days, walking 90 miles or more was very common. A two, three or four-day journey back then was the same as you and I hopping into our cars today and driving an hour and a half to work.

In biblical days, people simply didn't think twice about walking long distances, because walking was the most common means of transportation. There were no planes, trains, automobile, bicycles, skateboards, or mopeds. As a matter of fact, even though horses and donkeys were around, they were not used for daily transportation by the average person. So as you can see, our biblical brothers and sisters brothers and sisters got plenty of daily exercise through walking and by gathering and preparing their meals. They were exposed to the sun, the best source of vitamin D, yet skin cancer was nonexistent. In fact, I have aunts and uncles who grew up in the south some 70 to 80 years ago who were sharecroppers and worked in crop fields from sun up to sundown, day in and day out, year after year. Working in the heat and exposed to the sun, none of them ever developed skin cancer. Skin cancer involves more than just the pigmentation of your skin and sunscreen lotions. In tropical climates all around the world, people are constantly exposed to the sun without sunscreen protection, yet incidents of skin cancer are very rare. My point is our best source of Vitamin D comes from the sun, and actually provides protection from cancer. The problem today is we lay in the sun without being physically active, and without physical activity, our lymphatic system doesn't operate, affording us the ability to properly utilize this crucial vitamin that actually prevents cancer.

Notice I said that my relatives worked from sun up til sundown, the operative word here is worked. They constantly picked, pulled, hauled, and carried loads of farm products. They used various muscle groups all over their bodies, which forced their lymphatic system to constantly cleanse and recycle their blood. This removed waste and toxins through internal circulation and external perspiration. They didn't have the luxury of laying out in the sun, which worked to their advantage and probably saved their lives. This backbreaking work kept their lymphatic system healthy. There were no refrigerators to keep things from spoiling, so food gathering and preparation was a daily task. What's important to understand here is that this lifestyle kept them healthy because their bodies were constantly removing toxins and circulating nutrient-rich oxygenated blood throughout.

The bible teaches us that God gave mankind seed-yielding herbs and fruits for food, but he also commanded that they work in the garden as well. This combination of both mankind's diet, and working in the garden promoted health and longevity. Keeping humans physically active insured proper lymphatic circulation, which is missing in our culture today. This must have worked very well, because the patriarchs lived long, vibrant, healthy lives until the introduction of animal flesh into their diets.

Just as important as blood circulation is lymph fluid circulation. The lymphatic system is a complex network of thin vessels and organs. The function of the lymphatic system is really part of the immune system also. It helps to protect and maintain the fluid environment of the body by filtering waste from the blood, and producing white blood cells to fight off infection. Because these glands are located between various muscle groups throughout the body, they have to be squeezed by our muscles as we move in order to circulate this lymph fluid. I'll explain this more in detail later in the chapter. My point here is that proper health is tied to proper circulation which is absolutely tied to mobility and exercise. Today, too many believers don't incorporate exercise into their family's lives because they've misinterpreted one scripture. 1st Timothy 4:8, "For bodily exercise profits a little, but godliness is profitable for all things, having promise of the life that now is and of that which is to come.

Scripture misinterpretation is one of the leading causes of unnecessary sickness and death among believers today. In fact, it has been proven that people who make exercise a lifestyle habit look younger, healthier, suffer less illnesses, and actually live 15 to 25 years longer than those who don't. Now listen, if you're still not convinced, just look around you or visit any hospital, and you'll convince yourself. Our young people today, can barely run three miles without passing out or stopping every few yards to catch their breath. Now, we accept this as routine because we're out of shape and don't exercise ourselves. Listen, I don't care if it's just 15 minutes, turn off the TV, put the game controller down, and get up and exercise. If you're too tired after work, then go to bed 15 minutes earlier and wake up 15 minutes earlier to exercise.

Believers, I can't overstress the importance of making exercise a lifestyle habit. It's really a matter of life and death. Your physical well being is just as important as your spiritual well being. You must serve God with your whole mind, body, soul, and spirit. With the advantages we have today like transportation, refrigeration, and health clubs, you would think that we would be healthier. Actually, we would be healthier if it were not for two underlying issues, mainly, lack of exercise and a contaminated food supply. Lack of exercise is where we fall short, and the contaminated food supply is the tool the adversary uses to destroy the temple and our faith.

Believe me, if you are suffering physically, it will definitely have an impact on your spiritual well being. If your child becomes gravely ill, your spirit and possibly your faith will be adversely affected by this situation. Millions of parents miss church to take care of sick loved ones. It doesn't matter to Satan how you are defeated as long as you are defeated. He simply wants to keep you away from anything that has to do with God. Jesus made a very profound statement to His disciples telling them to live their lives by following after His examples. If Jesus and his disciples exercised, then it would behoove us to do the same.

It was about 24 years ago when I was told by friends, concerned for my health, that I should stop jogging so much. They were afraid I would damage my knees from the constant pounding on the concrete. I was warned that by the time I turned 30, my knees would be totally shot and I wouldn't be able to run at all. Well, I'm almost 40 years old, and thank God I didn't follow their advice and stop jogging. I still jog quite a bit, and in fact, sometimes I'll run up to 20 miles per week if I have time. I bring my four-year-old daughter along as I push her in her stroller on our scenic tour of rolling hills and lush green trees. What's amazing is the fact that my knees, or for that matter my entire body, has never felt better. As a matter of fact, I actually look forward to running more than I do sitting down to a meal. Running has become therapeutic, sort of like an outlet from all of the stresses and hassles of everyday life. I am able to worship the Father without any interferences. It's a really awesome experience.

I have been jogging every since I can remember, going all the way back to elementary school. It is my personal belief that the lifestyle changes I made earlier in life have had a major impact in regards to my health today. I talk to other people who are much older than I by some 30 to 40 years, and they also attribute their health and vitality to their healthier lifestyle habits. If you think you're too old or over the hill, guess what, you're not. An increasing number of studies continue to show that it is never too late to start exercising, and that even small improvements in physical fitness can significantly lower the risk of death. If you're out of shape or a couch potato, don't expect to go out and run in the Marine Corps Marathon. Begin with 15 to 20 minutes of light exercise or a brisk daily walk, and then gradually increase the intensity and duration of how long you exercise. Even after age 50, exercise can add healthy and active years to one's life.

Elderly people can prolong their lives and lessen their dependence of costly medications by simply walking regularly. People who are moderately fit even if they smoke or have high blood pressure have a lower mortality rate than the least fit. Elderly people can reduce loss of muscle mass through resistance exercises. Bone density, muscle mass, and strength can be maintained or even enhanced because these groups only respond to resistant training. Stiffness and loss of balance that accompanies aging can be greatly reduced by simply incorporating flexibility exercises.

Running does wonders for the body, enabling the body to become more oxygenated. The increased heart rate forces nutrient-rich, oxygenated blood, which rests deep in the bottom of the lung sacks, to be circulated throughout the body. This nutrient-rich blood can only be circulated through some type of aerobic exercise. It is amazing the number of believers who don't exercise, yet expect to miraculously maintain optimum health. Walking is one of the easiest and most beneficial exercises one can participate in. If you have children, it can be a lot of fun because the little ones love going outside. One can be totally healed of Type II diabetes simply by making routine exercise a part of their daily lives and changing a few unhealthy dietary habits.

As more and more cultures adopt western dietary habits, Type II diabetes particularly is reaching epidemic proportions throughout the world. Walking and other aerobic exercise is proving to have significant and particular benefits for people with both Type I and Type II diabetes. Regular exercise increases sensitivity to insulin, improves cholesterol levels, lowers blood pressure, and decreases body fat. In fact, older people who engage in regular exercise like walking briskly can lower their risk for diabetes without losing a pound. If you are taking insulin or suffering from diabetes, take special precautions before embarking on a workout program.

In the past decade, scientific evidence has shown that people who exercise not only live longer, they live better. Certain types of cancers, clogged arteries, diabetes, hypertension, and osteoporosis which are all associated with aging have been prevented through exercise. Numerous studies have shown that exercise training in coronary artery disease patients improves survival. Long-term exercise protects the blood vessels from changes related to aging and makes them more like those of a young person. Through exercise, the blood vessels of older people functioned just as well as those of younger people. Moderate exercise regularly reduces body fat, increases lean muscle, lowers blood pressure, drops insulin resistance, and raises HDL cholesterol, having a positive effect on the body overall.

Millions of Americans suffer from illnesses that can be prevented or improved through regular physical activity. Exercise is vital for proper circulation and maintaining overall health. Humans are not made to sit around for long periods and really, only in the past 100 to 150 years has the majority of the population been immobilized. Today between commuting back and forth to work, playing video games and watching TV, or sitting behind a desk, the average person gets very little physical activity. The whole body benefits from exercise including the heart, lungs, and muscles. This is because nutrient-rich blood is carried throughout the body and waste material is removed and forced out, keeping a proper balance. Increased circulation is the major benefit of exercise and better circulation is a major component to keeping healthy.

We need to exercise for two very important reasons, obviously good blood circulation, and also good lymph activity. I mentioned earlier that I would explain this more in detail. Just as important as blood circulation is lymph fluid circulation. Lymph fluid circulation is very important as it is the fluid other than blood contained in the tissues of the body. Lymph is a fluid made of digested proteins and fats, red blood cells, and many white blood cells, especially lymphocytes which attack bacteria in the blood. The lymphatic system is a network of vessels and nodes that transport the lymph throughout the body. The lymph glands are little nodules within the lymph vessels where white blood cells are made. The lymph glands are primarily located in your groin, throat, and armpits. The lymph system is a major component of the body's immune system. Lymph nodes produce immune cells such as lymphocytes, monocytes, and plasma cells. They also filter the lymph fluid and remove foreign material such as bacteria and cancer cells.

When bacteria are recognized in the lymph fluid, the lymph nodes enlarge as they produce additional white blood cells to help fight infection. Swelling and tenderness of the lymph glands is usually.

ally a good and bad sign. It is an indication that there is an infection somewhere near the swollen gland. This swelling and tenderness also indicates that the glands are working overtime to produce enough white blood cells to fight off the infection. Unlike the heart, the lymph glands must be squeezed by our muscles as we move in order to circulate the lymph fluid. Fortunately, this fluid can only travel through the cells in one direction and only by means of exercise.

It is important to understand the vital role that proper lymph circulation plays in maintaining optimum health. Blood circulation is completed through the lymph system. As the blood vessels get smaller and smaller, components of the blood are squeezed out through tiny spaces. Tissue fluid is excreted and carries nourishment to every cell in the body. Once the tissue fluid has passed on its nourishment, the lymph vessels will collect it up again. The fluid now also contains waste material, dead cells, and carbon dioxide. The lymph vessels then redirect the tissue fluid back towards the blood circulation system again, but only after the waste material is removed from it through the kidneys and liver. This is why it is imperative that the liver and kidneys stay healthy as they are very vital to keeping the body cleansed.

The lymph fluid has a vital task in transporting white blood cells around the body. White blood cells are the major component of our immune system. They immediately proceed to any area of damage or inflammation in the body. They fight off invading parasites, mutagent or cancerous cells, and repair or recycled damaged body cells coming to the end of their life cycle. The lymph vessels actually pass between the muscles of the body in many places. As muscles squeeze together, this action puts pressure on the lymph glands which pump the lymph fluid throughout the body. Without the lymph system working properly, the immune system is greatly compromised, which lessens the body's ability to fight off infection. This means that the body will not remove dangerous waste material nor will it circulate the army of white blood cells to fight off invaders. In other words, you have an army that cannot take the fight to the enemy because you're constantly sitting on your...well, you get the picture. This is why regular exercise is so important to making the lymph system work and keeping the body healthy. Otherwise, waste products build up in our bodies, and the white blood cells are not circulated to where they are needed.

Exercise is vitally important for diabetics, and it is imperative to the quality of their health. Nerve damage from diabetes is horrific causing blindness, loss of hearing, leading cause of kidney failure, and prevents healing when injuries occur. Blood sugar rises to 170 from a normal level of 110 after we eat. After reaching 170, the pancreas releases large amounts of insulin which causes blood sugar levels to fall. Diabetics either don't produce enough insulin or cannot respond adequately to this rise in blood sugar levels, so their blood sugar levels rise above 170. At this point, sugar attaches to cell membranes. Under normal conditions, sugar is harmless, but when it stays attached to cell membranes, it's converted into sorbitol, a toxic poison that causes tissue damage. It is this attachment of sorbitol to the nerve cells that causes nerve damage.

The liver and muscles remove sugar from the blood which keeps levels from rising too high after a meal, but only if they are empty of sugar. There is a limit as to the amount of sugar the liver and the muscles can retain. When you exercise, you empty blood sugars from your liver and muscles. After you eat again, sugar goes from your blood into the exercised muscles so blood levels do not rise too high. Watching sugar intake, but more importantly exercising can keep sugar levels in check preventing nerve cell damage and enabling the body to heal itself. The following precautions should be taken before starting an exercise program, especially if you are a diabetic. Don't exercise if your blood sugar is above 350. Make sure you eat first, take medications, and keep stevia, raisins, or honey around in case your blood sugar levels drop too low during exercise. Stevia is an excellent sweetener for diabetics because it's all natural and has no adverse affect on blood sugar levels. You may even want to consult with a personal trainer to make sure you get the proper amount of exercise.

An exercise program should start slowly and build up to more strenuous activities. The reduced risk of heart attack and death from heart attack is one of the greatest benefits of being physically active. For an overweight person, exercise is very important, as well as for anyone who has diabetes or other risk factors for heart disease. The Harvard Alumni study found that increased physical activity from 500 calories per week to 2,000 calories showed a reduction in death from heart attacks. Other studies from the Lipid Research Clinics found that men who were physically fit were less likely to die from heart attacks than men who were out of shape. Women over the age of 45 are equally at risk for a heart attack as men their age, because of the loss of protective hormones.

You can exercise without seeing a big difference in weight because when you exercise, you gain lean muscle which is heavier than fat. Exercise shouldn't be used solely to lose weight, but to change the condition of the body and make it healthier. People who exercise are more likely to maintain the weight they lose when compared to those who don't. In addition to increased energy levels, exercise increases nervous system activity and increases feelings of well being. You have a smaller chance of being depressed because of weight gain if you exercise.

The risk of developing the following diseases can be greatly reduced with routine exercise: premature death from heart disease, developing both Type I and II diabetes, developing high cholesterol, developing colon cancer, developing high blood pressure, developing breast cancer, developing depression and anxiety, developing osteoporosis, developing obesity. Regular exercise controls weight gain, builds and maintains healthy bones, muscles, and joints. It promotes psychological well-being, longevity, and improves quality of life. Exercise helps maintain full functioning and independence among the elderly. Physical activity reduces oxygen demand, the tendency for blood clots to form in arteries that have narrowed, and increases elasticity in the arteries. Women who suffer with difficult menstrual cycles can benefit greatly from routine exercise. The benefits of exercise far outweigh the benefits of not exercising. The duration and intensity of exercise should be gradually increased over time. Don't expect any overnight miracles as the benefits from exercise occur gradually and become evident over a one to two-month period. Also, exercise releases large amounts of the hormone dopamine into the bloodstream. With this hormone present, the feelings of hunger greatly diminish. This is an excellent way to manage your weight without starving yourself. It is also the healthiest approach to use, because it will actually strengthen and heal the body both inside and out. This is exactly why diet pills and gastric bypasses are not healthy approaches.

Exercise is half the battle. The other half is proper nutrition. You must honor God will all of your being and not just your spirit. He needs all of you so the Holy Spirit can continue the work of Christ here on the earth. The following is a chart showing the calories burned during certain types of exercises. This is not a complete list of all physical activities, but it will give you a little insight into what types of exercises you may want to be involved in. There is so much overwhelming evidence that proves beyond any doubt that a little exercise does profit the body a whole lot. If you intend to be around and in good health for a while, then you had better get busy. That's right. Start today. Get up right now. Don't wait for your friends. It's you and the Lord, and He's all you need. He promised to never leave nor forsake you as well as always watch over you. So just take comfort in knowing that even when you exercise, He is right there with you. **Remember, God has placed before you life and death, sickness and disease, so choose life, that you and your seed may live.**

Activity (1 hour)	135lbs	150lbs	195lbs
Aerobics general	350	418	500
Aerobics high impact	418	485	609
Aerobics low impact	270	380	440
Backpacking general	425	435	655
Basketball game	480	580	685
Basketball shooting baskets	286	325	398
Bicycling leisure	246	286	351
Bicycling light effort	364	438	525
Bicycling moderate	496	585	698
Bicycling vigorously general	595	746	875
Bicycling stationary light	290	360	440
Bicycling stationary moderate	413	493	604
Bicycling stationary very light	189	224	250
Bicycling stationary very vigorous	635	745	916
Boxing punching bag	365	430	535
Boxing sparring	540	645	786
Canoeing, rowing, crewing	754	824	1040
Canoeing rowing light	177	211	259
Dancing fast	354	422	518
Dancing slow	170	201	245

Activity (1 hour)	135lbs	150lbs	195lbs
Dancing general	266	317	358
Football touch	476	536	690
Football competitive	531	633	776
Golf general	236	281	355
Golf miniature	177	220	259
Handball general	710	875	1040
Jogging	413	419	604
Race walking	390	460	570
Racquetball	413	496	610
Rope jumping	710	850	1040
Running	238	883	1085
Running cross country	531	633	776
Running track	595	714	870
Running stairs	890	1060	300
Skating roller	420	495	610
Skating ice	540	640	740
Skiing cross country	535	635	780
Skiing general	420	500	615
Skiing water	360	425	535
Soccer	420	500	618
Softball	300	360	440
Swimming laps	560	650	750
Swimming backstroke	500	585	680
Swimming butterfly	650	784	951
Swimming leisurely	385	428	535
Swimming sidestroke	476	563	691
Swimming treading water	472	568	694
Tennis general	416	497	609
Volleyball	475	568	695
Walking	425	493	615
Walking Stairs	450	542	678
Walking uphill	358	426	528
Walking track	294	365	434
Water aerobics	240	285	349
Weight lifting	215	325	410

The calorie information listed on the previous pages are based on 1 hour of physical activity. Three separate categories are listed re-garding various weight classes. The numbers given may fluctuate up or down and are provided strictly for informational purposes only.

CHAPTER 14

Losing Weight Permanently

"I have set before you life and death, blessing and cursing: therefore choose life, that both thou and thy seed may live:" (Deuteronomy 30:19)

Last year, Americans spent some $45 billion on diet and weight loss products. Today, everywhere you look either someone is on a diet or about to start a new one. In fact, it seems that ever since I can remember, I've always known someone who was on some type of newly discovered diet, including myself, at one time or another. It seems as though people are really trying desperately to lose weight. Gaining weight is almost like getting cancer. So many people fear the thought of it that they remain nervously preoccupied with the dreadful idea that it might just happen. Last year, an astonishing $45 billion was spent just on diet products alone. Sadly, of all those people who spent $45 billion dollars to lose weight, more than two thirds wasted their hard earned money, because according to government studies, 65% of all dieters regain their weight back within one year. Further studies concluded that over a five-year period, 97% of all dieters regain all of their weight back and then some.

Let us stop here for a second and do the math: $45 billion x 5 years = $225,000,000,000. Probably a conservative half of that amount was spent by believers. Look at the staggering amount of wealth, $112,500,000,000, that was transferred out of the kingdom. Of course we really can't blame it all on Satan, because nothing he does can prosper without getting permission from ready and willing participants. Why are there so many people on diets in this country? Why do so many people go through all the trouble to lose weight, only to watch themselves regain it all back and then some? Why do so many people continually spend billions of their hard earned dollars, only to end up throwing it all away? Why do so many people devote so much of their precious time, effort, and energy, only to accomplish

191

dismal results? I don't care how you dice it or slice it, 97% is really just a complete failure. If you were hoping to graduate from college, but failed to pass 97% of the required curriculum, well you get the point. The fact is diet pills, videos tapes, CDs, books, pre-packaged meals, weight loss centers, and gastric bypass surgery, are simply not the answer. These approaches don't have the power to reach and effectively deal with the little person hiding on the inside of you.

You know the real you that no one really knows about except you. The you that stares back at you every time you look at yourself in the mirror. The you that you discuss your weight problem with, and then make promises about how you are going to change. The you that is inescapable just like your own shadow that follows you every where you go. There is nothing you can do to escape this you that talks back to you and says, "I really don't want to be overweight and obese, will you please help us?" The you that cries out when no one else is around, because your tired of fighting the bulge and wish there was an easier way out. The you when unseen and alone behind closed doors, places the diet on the night stand, and really gets down and pigs out. That's the real you that no diet pills, videos tapes, CDs, books, pre-packaged meals, weight loss centers, or gastric bypass surgery can change, the real you. Nor can they really change the underlying issues and conditions that are causing you to gain weight in the first place.

A close friend of mine once asked me to pray for his cousin who was gravely ill because she had overeaten one too many times, causing the staples in her stomach to rip apart. She had gotten her stomach stapled in order to lose weight and help control her problem with over-eating. Her medical approach to dieting failed, and now she was staring at death's door, because instead of making lifestyle changes, she took a short cut through medical surgery, which inadvertently led to her bleeding internally and becoming infected. The Apostle Paul tells us to be transformed by the renewing of our minds. Romans 12:2 says, "And do not conform to this world, but be transformed by the renewing of your mind, that you may prove what is that good and perfect will of God." It seems that she was able to transform her body, but her mind was really the key. I'm quite sure at some point she could feel the need to push away the plate, but decided to satisfy the desires of her flesh instead. The fact that her stomach had been stapled together proved that at some point, there was a conversation with the little person inside of her, and she had listened. It is the transforming of the real you in the mind that determines if your attempt to manage your weight will turn with out to be a true success or a complete failure.

If you notice, the cover of this books says *"this is not a diet but a lifestyle."* This statement is really where the true approach to managing your weight starts. Believers have fallen into the same trap as nonbelievers, and consequently speak the same language and use the same psychology when dealing with issues regarding weight control and obesity. Every believer should remove the word diet completely from their vocabulary as it relates to losing weight. The word diet is not mentioned one time in the entire Bible regarding managing and losing weight. It appears once in Jeremiah 52:33 where it speaks of the king of Babylon who released King Jehoiachin from prison and gave him regular daily portions all the days of his life. In fact, believers shouldn't be on diets to begin with, because weight management should be a natural part of their lifestyle. We don't go on spiritual diets to manage the sin in our lives. We make living holy a part of our daily lifestyle and use the word of God to guide us. We should approach managing our weight with the same type of lifestyle principals that we apply to our spiritual lives. If more people made weight management a lifestyle, losing weight would have a 97% success rate instead of the dismal failures we see repeated year after year.

Listen, I was once trapped too, going on diet after diet, always battling with myself trying to keep off the pounds, constantly seeking out the next new diet plan because the last five failed. It wasn't until I decided to stop dieting and make real lifestyle changes that I actually lost the weight and was able to keep it off. You see, I lost 50 pounds almost 20 years ago and never gained it back, all without the use of diet pills, weight loss videos or CDs, no Jenny Craig or Weight Watchers, and no surgical procedures. Once I stopped the dieting cycle and made weight management a part of my lifestyle, the weight just naturally dropped off effortlessly. Now the greatest benefits were not the pounds I was able to shed, but the internal cleansing and healing that actually took place. Instead of changing dietary habits and principals just to lose wight, it should become your lifestyle every minute of the day to improve the condition of your overall health.

Excess weight can lead to a lot other diseases like diabetes, hypertension, cancer, obesity, and heart disease. On the other hand, people who stay fit and healthy experience great health benefits and longevity. There are a lot of people who are fit but are not healthy, and that's the reason why lifestyle changes are far more important than just losing weight. One of the natural by-products of using the life-style approach is that weight loss comes naturally and effortlessly. There are many factors that contribute to weight gain, but there are only two real reasons why one gains weight in the first place. They are the unlimited availability of all kinds of foods 24 hours a day, and the unhealthy lifestyle choices people often make. If you were to hop on an airplane and travel to any poor and starving third world country where there are famished people who don't have access to food 24 hours a day, there would be one common scene that encompasses every continent you travel to. The primary overwhelming scene would be one of many thin-framed, underweight people, and the complete absence of overweight or obese people. In fact, if you did happen to see someone standing around weighing 300 or more pounds amongst millions of skinny, almost skeletal looking starving people, they would look quite awkward and immediately stand out like a sore thumb. The news media would give more attention to this one obese 300-pound person than the millions of other people starving to death.

No, for some unknown reason, millions of starving people who don't have access to food 24 hours a day look pretty much in the same condition, underweight and suffering with malnutrition. There are no weight loss centers, no pre-packaged, reduced-calorie, low-fat meals, no diet pills, or fat removal clinics. This brings me to my next point. In countries where people have access to food 24 hours a day, just the opposite happens. Everyone is either overweight or obese. Look at America for instance, the land of good and plenty anytime you want it. We have grocery stores, fast food restaurants, donut shops, and vending machines operating 24 hours a day just to feed us whenever we get hungry.

I read an article recently in the paper about a 42-year-old man living in the mid-west who weighed an astonishing 1,097 pounds standing at just under 6 feet tall. His more than half-ton body caused him to lose his mobility and he could no longer walk. He also developed life-threatening medical complications that included heart disease, hyper-tension, diabetes, and shortness of breath. Dr. Xavier Pisunyer, an obesity expert at Columbia University in New York, says "people with excess fat tend to have higher free fatty acids circulating in the blood." "There has been some data to suggest that higher circulating free fatty acids could be a risk factor for increased cardiac arrhythmia," Pi-Sunyer said. This man was dying because he chose not to live by healthy lifestyle principals.

Before becoming disabled, he worked long hours as a manager in the food and restaurant business, and had access to food whenever he wanted to eat. So he eventually ate himself into disability 16 years ago, and although he could no longer work or walk, he continued eating until he had grown to more than a half-ton in weight. You would expect a person eating so much food to be well-nourished, but believe it or not, he was actually suffering from malnutrition, because all of his calories came from foods high in fat and carbohydrates. He was placed on a special scale used to weigh trucks loaded with grain to determine his weight. A specially equipped ambulance with a heavy-duty stretcher, winches, ramps and other tools carried him to the hospital, after an exterior section of wall was removed from his house. I want you to understand something. He didn't just happen to gain 1,000 pounds overnight. For many years, he had access to food 24 hours a day, at work and at home, and all of the food stops in between. The problem is he never held himself accountable for his own bad eating habits. I know you're asking yourselves why didn't someone intervene and try to save him earlier in his life. Actually, he tried saving himself for many years, constantly using different types of diets plans, but eventually admitted that every diet he ever tried always failed. He had struggled with weight problems since kindergarten where he weighed 90 pounds, and had reached 250 pounds by the time he was in middle school. He also probably inherited some bad eating habits passed down from his father and grandfather who both weighed more than 300 pounds each.

Fortunately, by the time I had started writing this book, he had managed to lose over 400 pounds. He finally realized that if he was going to save his life and live, he had to implement some healthy lifestyle changes. This man is not alone. Over 100,000 people are morbidly obese in this country. Now for some unknown reason, almost 70% of this nation's population is either overweight or obese. With all the new diet products, self-help books, weight loss centers, and advances in surgical procedures available today, from the least to the greatest, people are still continuing to pack on the pounds. Some have even been misguided into believing that they suffer with some type of medical disorder that causes them to just naturally gain an extra 150 to 200 pounds. Government studies have proven that only a very tiny fraction of the general population in this country suffers from such disorders. In other words, if you were dropped off in a poor third-world country and lacked access to food, you would look just like the local starving people around you. It might take a few weeks or maybe even a couple of months, but if all you had to eat every day was a bowl of steamed rice, you would shed the pounds as well. Most people who think they suffer with some type of medical weight gain condition really don't. This takes us back to the previous point. In starving countries that don't have access to food 24 hours a day, issues related to weight control and obesity are non-existent.

Now am I telling you to go out and starve yourself? Of course not. Now I want you to get a clear picture as to what is causing the spiraling out of control epidemic of weight gain and obesity in this country. Our children are swollen and uncomfortable looking as they struggle to lug around excess weight. You can't go shopping without seeing someone driving themselves around inside the store. So many people are suffering with debilitating medical conditions that are directly linked to their unhealthy lifestyles. Again, in my opinion, there are only two reasons why people can't control their weight in this country. With these two reasons are a myriad of extenuating influences and factors that greatly contribute to both the physical and psychological causes. These influences and factors cause a lot of confusion by clouding and complicating the two main reasons. This explains why 97% of all dieters fail miserably at controlling their weight, and within five years not only regain the original weight they initially lost, but a whole lot more.

Having access to food 24 hours a day and choosing not to follow healthy lifestyle principals are the two main causes of obesity and weight loss failures in this country. Before the use of debit cards and ATM machines became widely available, people had access to to money only during normal banking ours. Today, with 24-hour ATM machines, people have unlimited access to money, so consequently, they spend a lot more. Look at the invisible link between the increase in debit card use and the increase in overweight people. More access equals more usage. Either way, having more may not always be the best option. Think about this for a minute. Back in biblical days, food had to be planted, grown and ripened, then harvested before it could be eaten. There were no food processing plants or any 24-hour diners. No McDonald's, Burger King, Taco Bell, Wal-Mart, or 7-11. People didn't have the luxury of refrigerators, stoves, or microwave ovens. Unlimited access to food 24 hours a day simply wasn't possible, because there was no way of preserving it or keeping it fresh. People didn't have food laying around for three or four weeks without it spoiling. They ate what they cooked and they made the next meal fresh.

Now I know you can't force the restaurants in your neighborhood to stop operating 24 hours a day so you don't have access. Listen, you can make mental lifestyle changes and not allow the food to have access to you by simply changing the types of food you consume and the times of day you allow yourself to eat. Some people won't eat pass 6 pm or they only eat certain types of food. So much of the food we eat today is specifically produced to make us like it and want more of it, even if it is totally unhealthy. Because of the adversary's influence and the love of money driving these giant food conglomerates, your health and safety is pushed aside for their profits.

For instance, everybody knows that sugar really isn't good for you. You've heard it ever since you were a toddler from your parents and grandparents. The food industry knows that sugar is bad for you too, but they also know that without sugar, many customers won't buy their products. Without customers, there is really no reason to be in business. That's why almost everything you buy is loaded with sugar, and just because it doesn't say the word sugar, doesn't mean it doesn't contain sugar. There are all kinds of chemical derivatives of sugar like high fructose corn syrup, potassium sorbate, sodium erthrobate, saccharin, aspartame, Splenda, neotame, acesulfame, sucralose, sucrose, maltose, maltodextrin, dextrose, sorbitol, corn syrup, barley malt, and caramel just to name a few. All of these sugars are a health hazard to the human body because most of them are chemi-cal drugs, and they are consumed in very large quantities. So every believer should throw out the diet products, especially the diet sodas, because believers shouldn't be on diets in the first place.

Remember, we're still primitive as it relates to how our bo-dies function. The way our bodies break down food and digest it hasn't changed much since biblical days. The big difference between back then and now is the fact that they ate whole foods like complex carbohydrates, grains, lean meats, poultry, fish, and drank water, na-turally sweetened fruit juice, or wine. They were also physically ac-tive in that they had to harvest their own foods, and walked almost everywhere. Today, our diets mainly consist of empty foods (refined white sugar, flour and pasta,) loaded with artificial sweeteners that are highly toxic to the body. For instance, drinking more than one can of soda per day can increase your chances of gaining weight by 80%.

Just look at aspartame, which has had more complaints than any other food additive. It has been implicated in causing lupus, multiple sclerosis, fibromyalgia, headaches, migraines, panic attacks, central nervous disorders, dizziness, gas, nausea, irritability, intestinal discomfort, skin rashes, nervousness, cramping, depression and manic episodes, male infertility, bloating, insomnia, mood swings, insulin imbalances, obesity, and inflamation. In the same way that no artifi-cial sacrifice could atone for the sin of mankind, no artificial sub-stance can take the place of real food. For instance, saccharin was proven to cause bladder cancer in laboratory rats. So the USDA re-quired warning labels be placed on all food products containing this carcinogen. Yet believers and non-believers alike bought and con-sumed products containing saccharin. Saccharin is now being re-placed buy a new chemical sweetener called Splenda. Every time your diet includes these substances, you are defiling the temple of God. 1st Corinthians 3:17 says, "If anyone defiles the temple of God, God will destroy him. For the temple of God is holy." Which temple are you.

If you compare the huge increases in sugar in our diets over the past century, particularly in processed foods, it matches succinct-ly in line with the precipitous rise in obesity and the epidemic in-creases of metabolic diseases. The average American now consumes about 130 pounds of sugar per year. That's more than forty teaspoons of sugar for every man, woman and child, every day, 365 days per year. The recommended consumption of sugar by the USDA is an average of no more than 10 teaspoons a day for a healthy adult which, in my opinion, is still too much, especially for women who are more adversely affected by sugar than men. Most of our toddlers and young children surpass the USDA recommendations by noon time. To make matters worse, concerned parents add a sugary fruit drink instead of water to their children's lunches. The biggest sources of artificial sweeteners are the corn sugars and high fructose corn syrups found in beverages like fruit juices and soda.

Sugar is a food processor's dream, because it's so cheap, adds flavor and texture, and makes consumers prefer their product over a less sweet alternative. So today, consumers get sugar in just about everything they buy, from simple carbohydrates like refined white granulated sugar, to more complex chemical poisons that include dextrose, high fructose corn syrup, maltodextrin, Splenda, and a host of other artificial sweeteners. These chemical sweeteners are just empty calories that take the place of real nutrients. So while we eat and pack on the pounds, we are really starving our cells and they began to mutate and regenerate into diseased cells. Without new healthy cells, the cell tissues that makes up our vital organs can't replace the spent and dying cells. Now our organs become handicapped, trying to function properly with new cell replacements that are diseased. This process begins the catastrophic degenerative decline in the quality of your health. Our entire digestive process is thrown completely out of kilter, and uncontrollable weight gain kicks in. In other words, our cells simply go crazy from the lack of proper balancing of nutrients in the same way society has gone crazy by lacking proper nutrients.

The disproportionate use of artificial sweeteners including refined sugar in the foods we eat, combined with mineral-depleted salt that prevents proper digestion, and the lack of fiber in our diets is directly proportionate to the number of people struggling to control their weight, and fighting to prevent the current obesity epidemic. This same condition of our food supply also reflects the increase in people suffering from mental illness and committing violent crimes. What's the major problem? We have access to the wrong kinds of food 24 hours a day every day of the year, which is over saturation. Refined sugar added to any diet, even in small amounts, is unhealthy because it causes your food to spoil in your stomach. After the food spoils, the body tries to pass it out. Any food that is not passed out is stored in the body as excess fat. So people go on yo-yo diets, removing sugary foods, and lose weight only to gain it all back once these type of foods are reintroduced back into their diets.

Because they haven't connected their weight to what they eat mentally, and haven't made the necessary lifestyle changes, they will continue to yo-yo with disappointing results. Losing weight and keeping it off is actually not that difficult at all. I have maintained my current weight for the past 20 years. I eat whenever I want, any time night or day, but I don't eat whatever I want. There are certain foods that I no longer consider real food, so I don't include them as part of what I eat. The rest of this chapter will deal with what you will need to do in order to lose weight permanently and improve your overall health. You are guaranteed to shed the pounds and keep them off by adhering to the rest of the information provided in this chapter.

Remember, you were not born overweight or obese. These conditions manifested over time as you consumed more and more of the wrong types of foods. Also, no two people are born exactly the same or have the same body chemistry. So don't compare the amount of time it takes you to lose weight with somebody else. There are many factors that come into play, to include how you were raised, and to what extent you participated in the unhealthy habits. Simply keep your eyes on yourself and let the other person watch themselves. I promise, you will be pleasantly surprised with your results if you concentrate on yourself and stay consistent. I'll repeat that again. Keep your eyes on yourself and stay consistent. You must not totally give up or stop because you lose 10 or 15 pounds. Even if you don't try everyday, do not totally give up.

How to lose weight and keep it off permanently? The first step to losing weight permanently is to start eating more whole foods that contain natural fiber, minerals, nutrients, and are not commercially processed. These types of foods burn faster so the body doesn't get the chance to store them as fat. Eating lots of organic foods whenever possible, fruits, vegetables, salads, whole grains, nuts, seeds, beans, and lean meats like fish and poultry is very beneficial. Eating other meats should be limited to once or twice a month. All seafood should be avoided because they are highly toxic and high in choles-

terol. All poultry should be boiled first to remove most of the hormones, antibiotics, pus, and other contaminates. This also will reduce the amount of fat and cholesterol in the meat itself. Boiling has
always been a means of purification even in biblical days. Remove
the skin from your poultry as it is high in fat. You can also bake the
chicken after you boil it. When it is done boiling, lightly cover it with
olive oil, herbal seasonings, and black pepper. Add sea salt in moderation and eat as much as you like along with all the vegetables
you want, and be happy.

My aunt, who is almost 80, has been eating her poultry this
way for the past twenty-five years. She was starting to gain a lot of
weight and decided to make lifestyle changes. I can honestly say that
since she made this change, she has never struggled with her weight
or suffered with any type of degenerative disorder. If it worked for
her, it will certainly work for you. Today, at almost 82 years of age,
she is active and vibrant, she doesn't use a cane, is not taking medications, and is not crippled over. She has some issues regarding memory loss, but other than that, she appears to be fine. As your body
restores its balances of minerals, you will start gaining more control
of your weight management problem. With a proper mineral balance,
you'll have proper digestion, which will result in your food breaking
down into the proper sugars from which we get the proper energy to
fuel our bodies.

While your body cannot survive without fat, 90% of your daily
intake of fat should solely come from extra virgin cold pressed olive
oil in its raw natural state. Moderate amounts of olive oil may even
reduce abdominal fat if eaten as part of a diet high in plant foods.
Olive oil is a mono-unsaturated fat that is easily and readily assimilated in the body. Research has shown people who use olive as their
primary source of fat have an overall balanced distribution of body
fat, and actually lose weight easier than people on low-fat, high-
carbohydrate diets. Also, olive oil adds a lot of zest and robust flavor
to your foods. Drinking eight to twelve glasses of water a day is important for anyone trying to lose weight. Water is used by the body
to flush and cleanse your cells. Weight loss can be greatly optimiz-
ed by drinking lots of water, even up to a gallon a day.

A total body detox should be started immediately and a complete liver detox may additionally be needed. The liver is a major fat

burning organ, and it pumps excess fat out of the body through the bile into your gut. A common problem with people who find it hard losing weight is a disease called NASH, where the liver is being over saturated with fat and loses its ability to function properly. Under normal conditions, the liver will burn and remove fat from the body. In fact, the liver is the highest fat burning organ in the body. However, when NASH sets in, this condition clogs the liver with unhealthy excess fat, so it can't burn nor remove fat from the blood. Weight loss becomes very difficult if not all but impossible. Weight will normally collect around the upper and lower abdomen. This condition affects both young and old with devastating consequences if not properly treated. People who have this disease normally suffer with diabetes and autoimmune diseases. However, a complete liver detox will get the liver functioning properly again. Avoiding all dairy foods is very important in reversing this condition and is beneficial for anyone attempting to lose weight.

Don't believe the hype on television commercials touting milk as a great weight loss product. If you notice, the person in the commercial is not struggling with a weight problem. They're slim and petite. The less dairy you consume, the more lean muscle mass you can maintain. Most dairy products are loaded with sugar, fat, mineral-depleted salt, and artificial sweeteners. Some people try to get by on a low-fat or fat-free diet, but as a I stated before, the human body needs fat to function properly, so a fat-free diet is very unhealthy. It's not so much the fat itself, but the type of fat. Also remember that heating or burning fat especially at high temperatures will greatly degrade and alter the molecular structure of the fat. Low-fat dairy products are loaded with sugar or artificial sweeteners, even though they may not appear on the label. If you do consume dairy products, make sure to drink plenty of lemon water with it. The acid in lemons is very powerful in breaking down fat while the water continuously flushes your body.

Separation of food types and proper food combination is vitally important and imperative to weight management. All proteins (meats, poultry, fish, eggs, dairy, nuts, beans, etc.) should be eaten separately from all starches (potatoes, pasta, rice, bread, etc.) Two different types of enzymes are used in the stomach to break down food. When these enzymes come in contact with each other, they cancel each other out. This action causes your food to spoil in your stomach with some of it ultimately being stored as fat. In order for your food to be properly broken down and assimilated, it must be fully digested first. It is important that foods be eaten in their proper combinations. The only thing you should drink with any meal is purified or distilled water. All other sugary drinks should be consumed by themselves or totally avoided. Medications are toxic to the body, especially the liver and kidneys, and are known to contribute to weight gain. People who take medicine regularly have a harder time losing weight. Also, the body will body will retain more water when medications are present because of their toxicity.

Exercise of any type, especially brisk walking, jogging, jump roping, or swimming are very beneficial to weight loss and overall body wellness. It doesn't matter if you exercise for 20 minutes or an hour, or two to four times per week, just as long as you exercise. I like to do a workout routine I've developed when I don't have time to get out and run. I begin by doing jumping jacks for five minutes, followed by three sets each of 100 sit ups and 30 push ups. Now of course if you are just starting out, you want to go easy depending on your size and abilities.

You might want to start off with just five minutes of jumping jacks at a moderate pace, and increase your pace as you lose weight. Add to this three sets each of 25 sit-ups and 15 push ups. Gauge yourself and see how you feel, as I wouldn't recommend overdoing it starting out. Make sure to use some type of shock absorbing pad while doing jumping jacks to limit excess stress and injury to the knees and ankles. Stretching is very effective in conjunction with exercise and proper nutritional habits. If jumping jacks are too difficult initially, try walking briskly for 15 minutes along with the sit ups and push ups. As you lose weight, you will be able to add more demanding exercises. Avoid fried foods and breads unless they are baked at home, or are organic whole grain from a health food store. Eat the bread with your vegetable meal only if you must have bread. Beans, apples, and raw garlic are really effective in curbing hunger. Eat whole grains for breakfast instead of precessed cereals. Replace all sweeteners with stevia, honey, black strap molasses, or pure maple syrup. Use olive oil instead of butter or margarine, you'll love the taste. Replace table salt and seasoning salts with Celtic Sea Salt.

Don't listen to all the commercials you hear about weight loss and dairy or the latest clinical study, because eventually they all change and people still have problems managing their weight.

Moderation and whole unprocessed foods are the only methods that really work. The advantage this approach has over traditional dieting is that this program actually heals the body. So you can also recover from diabetes, hypertension, heart disease, obesity, and certain types of cancer. Studies have proven that obese people are more susceptible to certain types of cancers. Don't expect results overnight and don't be too anxious. It took time to gain weight, and it will take time to lose it. I don't like using scales, because they can complicate matters by not showing the numbers one would like to see. Remember, as you replace fat with lean muscle mass, lean muscle weighs more than fat so the scale may not move much. Instead of seeing a dramatic drop in weight, you may notice a leaner, toner, body.

I personally allow my body weight to fluctuate between five to ten pounds in either direction. I think this is healthy, because it keeps me from panicking and worrying about my weight, as worry and excess stress can also complicate weight management. In addition, plus five or ten pounds for an active person is very easy to burn off. So I leave myself this little extra cushion and so far, it has worked very effectively. Exercise will help keep the hormone dopamine in the blood, which will greatly help curb uncontrollable hunger urges. Listen, I am no different than any of you. I grew up eating all the wrong foods which I was led to believe were healthy. If I can lose weight and keep it off, so can you. We are no different. A lifestyle change combined with consistency is all that it takes. This approach will work, I promise it will, as long as you do your part. **Remember, God has placed before you life and death, sickness and disease, so choose life, that you and your seed may live.**

C H A P T E R 15

Natural Remedies
for Common Ailments

"I have set before you life and death, blessing and cursing: therefore choose life, that both thou and thy seed may live:" (Deuteronomy 30:19)

When the Twin Towers were struck on 911, the buildings burned for quite some time before finally collapsing and falling down to the ground. The fires overwhelmed the structural integrity of the buildings, and in the absence of overwhelming force to put them out, the fires were able to burn out of control and overtake the towers. Fire and acidity are analogous in the way in which they cause destruction. Both use heat to destroy whatever they come in contact with. A fire can start in one room, and if not immediately brought under control, will spread to other rooms of a house. However, if the other rooms are saturated with water, the fire will have a much harder time spreading. Water is full of oxygen, the main fuel for fire, so you would think that the fire would have an easier time spreading. However, because each oxygen atom in water is surrounded by two hydrogen atoms, the extra hydrogen atoms actually protect the other saturated rooms from the fire and prevents the fire from spreading with ease.

This is what happens in the amniotic sac of the mother's womb. The presence of extra hydrogen atoms protects the fetus from acidity and bacteria, as it develops in the mothers whom. This balanced matrix of hydrogen and oxygen in our blood protects our cells from the same conditions. When this delicate balance is altered for an extended period of time, degenerative diseases start to develop. In the same way that they are developed, they must be reversed in order for the body to heal itself and totally recover from these life threatening conditions. Remember, the purpose of changing your nutritional lifestyle is not to lose weight, but to create a healthier you from the inside out. The following list of common ailments are just a few of many that are plaguing our society today. Just about every common ailment has two factors involved: what we allow to enter our bodies and how we remove toxic waste from our bodies.

When your clothes need cleaning, you buy laundry detergent to wash them. We''re so concerned about how clean we are on the outside while we are rotting on the inside. Some of our bodies on the inside look and smell like a garbage landfill. We have parasites and disease hovering all around our cells, and without any type of cleansing, our cells become a part of the decaying, putrefying landscape. Eventually, because our entire bodies are made up of living cells, we start to physically look on the outside like what's taking place on the inside. You must consistently cleanse your inner terrain through what you eat, exercise, with distilled water, and by various forms of detoxification. Mineral-rich foods and soils are imperative to the survival of this nation. Both degenerative diseases and crime are escalating as IQ and nutritional status deteriorate. These conditions are inextricably connected and the end cause is impoverishment of the soil.

For certain diseases not covered in this section, please feel free to email questions concerning your condition to sales@blessand-eat.com.

The following steps should be taken in reversing and preventing the all following conditions:

Exercise: 30-45 minutes of brisk walking, jogging, or bicycle riding.
Detox & Cleansing: Total body cleanse, Parasitic cleanse, Candida cleanse.
Daily Detox: ½ fresh squeezed lemon, distilled water, 3 to 4 shakes Celtic salt, and stevia (diabetic friendly), ½ Tsp Cayeen pepper
Garlic: Fresh organic garlic
Follow Daily Meal Planner: Chapter 6
Remove: Hydrogenated oils; margarine; table salt; refined sugar; soft drinks; coffee; non-organic dairy products, especially milk and products containing milk; commercial white flour and processed wheat products; totally eliminate canned foods. (expt. some organic products)
Add: extra virgin, 1st cold pressed olive oil, flaxseed oil, Smart Balance buttery spread, Celtic Salt, stevia, honey, maple syrup, black strap mo-

lasses, frozen vegetables (organic) or Hanover brands, herbs, whole wheat (unprocessed).

Heal and Prevent Diabetes

Type I and II diabetes are both reversible, even if there is a family history of these conditions. Normally, sugar is stored in the liver and muscles until it is needed. When you exercise, the body empties this storage of sugar into the blood to be used for energy. When the liver and muscles empty out this storage of sugar, they are now ready to store more sugar. When you eat, your blood sugar levels immediately rise from 120 to around 170. At this point, the pancreas releases insulin to prevent sugar levels from rising above 170 and staying there for too long. To do this effectively, the liver and muscles must be regularly emptied of sugar. If not, sugar builds up in the body and sugar levels become difficult to maintain and control. This is why exercise is so important because it keeps the body from storing too much sugar. Your body turns refined sugar into five times more fat in the blood than starches. A loss of just 5% to7% in body weight can reverse Type II diabetes.

The average daily meals we consume consist of too much sugar and not enough green vegetables or fiber to balance out the meal. Also hydrogenated oils adversely affect the beta cells which are responsible for the production of insulin. The good thing is that over time, with healthier nutritional habits, diabetes can be reversed and healed. Remember, one must be very careful when eating processed foods, because they are loaded with sugar, sodium, trans fats, and thousands of artificial toxic substances. It is imperative for diabetics to eat a lot less cooked foods and more fresh, raw foods. Foods that cook for long periods start to caramelize and this action has an adverse affect on blood sugar levels.

Add: 2 apples and ½ cup of beans daily (black, kidney, or chic peas).

Herbs: Atractylodis, Garlic, Ginseng, Green tea, Fenugreek, Burdock

Heal and Prevent Hypertension

Keeping blood pressure under control is not as hard as one would think. Refined salt and sugar are major contributing factors, along with obesity, smoking, and other unhealthy generational habits. This condition worsens as toxic table salt forces the body into survival mode. Table salt has a high concentration of sodium, which is highly explosive and over-acidifies the body. Acid is corrosive and burns, so when this happens, our cells use excess water in our bodies for protection. This defensive mechanism causes blood pressure to rise and can be catastrophic depending on the condition of the arteries and blood vessels. Exercise and nutritional habits are very instrumental if one is to manage this condition effectively. Try to buy reduced sodium or sodium-free foods and season the food yourself with Celtic Sea Salt. Celtic Sea salt in conjunction with water can actually help regulate blood pressure.

Remember, a salt-free diet is dangerous and can be deadly to your health. You need salt, but absolutely stay away from refined table salt. Only use a salt that has been tested for full mineral content like Celtic Sea Salt, which in conjunction with water, can actually help to regulate blood pressure. This condition is definitely linked to poor nutritional habits and lack of exercise. Just making a conscious decision to avoid certain types of foods, especially pork and products containing high amounts of sodium, is vitally important. High blood pressure can lead to other types of degenerative diseases. Sugar also has an affect on blood pressure, so try to use all-natural sweeteners.

Follow Daily Meal Planner: Add figs, kiwi, prunes, dates, grapes, raisins, foods that are rich in potassium.

Herbs: Ginseng, Dong Quai, Hawthorn, Bilbery, Scutellaria, Garlic

Heal and Prevent Heart Disease

This condition has a myriad of contributing factors that accumulate over time. Heart disease takes years to develop and manifest. The major problem with this disease is that most often the manifestations are sudden and without advance warning. This is why prevention is the ultimate insurance policy for this particular deadly disease. One out of every two women die from heart disease every year. Fortunately, this condition is reversible and is definitely preventable. Unhealthy fats, cholesterol, commercially-processed milk and dairy products, acidic conditions of the blood, smoking, and lack of exercise are all major contributing factors and greatly complicate this disease. The average American diet has been almost completely void of essential fatty oils like omega 3, 6, and 9 EFAs. Essential fats are fats that the body needs but cannot produce on its own.

They have to be supplemented from sources outside the body. We use to get these oils from our consumption of animal meats that were raised on green vegetation, but with the introduction of hydrogenated oils and grain fed animals, we no longer receive healthy amounts of essential fats in our diets. These fats are vitally important to all body functions, especially the heart. Table salt possesses other dangers, because it lacks the proper minerals that the heart requires to maintain healthy. Minerals are needed to help regulate heart rhythm and gently keep the arteries and blood vessels clear of plaque. Milk and dairy products scar the artery walls and over time, leads to build up and blockage of the blood vessels. Flax seeds are our best source of EFAs, along with fish oils. Avoid fried foods, smoking, and processed dairy products.

Follow Daily Meal Planner: Add flax seed oil and ground flax seed; fish and fish oils are also good supplements; extra virgin olive oil.
Herbs: Garlic, Bitter Orange, Turmeric, Astragalus

Heal and Prevent Cancer

Cancer is simply a condition resulting from mutagent cells that overtake the entire body causing disruption and suppression of system functions. These cells thrive in an acidic and oxygen-deprived environment. All cell function ceases when the condition of the blood is either too alkaline or too acidic. In the same way, a healthy person will die if their body temperature goes below or above a certain level. The American diet for the past 70 years has been mostly acidic due to processed foods that are preserved with refined sugar, refined salt, and hydrogenated oils. Not to mention that they are totally void of real nutrition. This situation over acidifies the blood which takes the body's pH dangerously out of balance. Without a balance of natural alkaline foods like fruits, vegetables, and herbs to oxygenate the blood, our cells will die.

Cancer shows up as a tumor which is really just entombed mutagent and dead cells, excess acids, and other toxins collected from the blood and deposited into the body's weakest areas. The internal organs that cleanse the body could not remove the excessive acid fast enough. This acidic condition lowers the amount of available oxygen in the blood leading to cell degeneration and eventually cell death. These degenerative cells and acid start attaching to healthy cells and begin to adversely affect them. This causes a domino affect and is where the process of cancer starts. Oxygen deprivation leads to cell asphyxiation, and dead cells in the blood cause an acidic build up. This acid impairs and destroys other healthy cells, and causes electrical cellular disturbances. As this situation of premature cell death continues, our healthy bacteria is transformed into unhealthy yeast, fungus and molds that produce toxic waste matter. In the absence of oxygen, sugar ferments. Also be advised that sugar, fat, and cholesterol feed cancer. The growth of cancer starts by the process of fermentation which can only take place in the absence of oxygen. In the absence of oxygen, carbon dioxide builds up as acidic waste. When blood pH falls below seven, oxygen is cut off and coma and death soon follow. The pH level of the blood is like that of our body's temperature, in that both must maintain a healthy balance. The pH of the blood should be maintained at around 7.30-7.40. In an extended acidic condition, the cells that don't die mutate into dangerous abnormal yeast cells which become malignant. Cancerous cells lack the DNA codes of normal healthy cells, thus they don't follow instructions and continue to multiply indefinitely and totally out of order. According to scientific research, flax seed oil has been proven to shrink tumors by up to 50% and pomegranate juice by up to 85%. Additional experiments on cultured human prostate cells showed that pomegranate juice inhibited cell growth.

Follow Daily Meal Planner: Add grapefruit seed extract, grape seed extract, pomegranate juice, flax seed oil.

Herbs: Garlic, Cat's claw, Quercetin

Heal and Prevent HIV/AIDS

This disease for the most part is preventable through lifestyle choices and behavioral changes. Sexual promiscuity is the leading cause for the spread of this disease. Homosexual men are affected by this disease far greater than any other sector of society. The second group of people affected by this disease are drug abusers. Last year, 3 million people died from AIDS and every day it takes another 8,200 lives. Air can kill the virus, which can live for up to six weeks in a syringe. This viral infection weakens the immune system causing the body to become susceptible to a host of other diseases. Because most people born in this country suffer with immune dysfunction most of their lives anyway, this virus has the ability to easily overtake the body. The American diet is too poor in nutrition and actually destroys a person's immune system because it is extremely over processed and stripped of all disease-fighting minerals, vitamins, and nutrients. The best way to combat this disease is through abstinence for those who are not married. If you are married, having sexual intercourse only with your spouse is definitely advised. If you are already diagnosed with the disease, you should follow the previous two recommendations along with a change in how you eat and prepare your foods. All cooked foods should be boiled before eating. Your meals should represent a 85% raw and 15% cooked mix. Also, these meals should include slightly more alkaline food groups found in **Chapter 6**. Garlic, ginseng, Celtic Sea salt, grapefruit seed and grape seed extract, flaxseed oil, extra virgin olive oil, and plenty of exercise are all needed to bring this condition under control. Avoid all sugar and artificial sweeteners, trans-fats or hydrogenated oils, refined foods, alcohol, smoking, and tap water. This is the only disease where I truly recommend that you absolutely boil all of your meats, and your fish should be only organic.

Follow Daily Meal Planner: flaxseed oil, grapefruit and grape seed extract.

Herbs: Aloe, Garlic, Cat's claw, Licorice, Rooibos, Maitake

Heal and Prevent Premature Aging

There are three things that promote premature aging: lack of proper rest, sugar, and cooked foods. This explains why the patriarchs lived with such longevity. They had no refined sugar, no artificial light, and only ate raw foods. Raw foods naturally slow the progress of aging because they contain living enzymes that lessen the stress of digestion on the body. Also heat kills vital nutrients, vitamins, and minerals needed to cleanse and repair cells. Cooking at temperatures above 130° Fahrenheit changes the molecular structure of all foods in pretty much the same way that burning your skin produces a different look and texture. Tests have proven that this change is a major factor behind many degenerative diseases because of excess free radicals present in the blood. Rest is very important because this is when the body replenishes itself and repair cells. Sugar is one of the highest acidifying substances and it stresses out every cell and organ in the body. Heat causes foods to produce high amounts of advanced glycation end products (AGEs), which are toxic and can cause cells to produce proteins that cause inflammation. There is no fountain of youth to prevent premature aging. However, there are three definite things one can do to slow its progression. Get plenty of rest, avoid sugar to include non-fruit based starches, and eat a diet of 85% raw and 15% cooked foods.

Heal and Prevent Ulcers

This condition is a result of acidic erosion in the lining of the stomach. It is an open wound that forms in the stomach or small intestine. For almost 100 years, doctors believed they were caused by stress, spicy foods and alcohol, but recent medical research has revealed that most ulcers are caused by a bacterial infection resulting from certain medications and smoking. The average American diet consists of foods that are highly acidic through frying, barbequing, and baking. This constant acidic diet further complicates ulcers, because bacteria thrive in an acidic oxygen-deprived environment. It is interesting to note that few people are born with this condition, but many develop it as they get into early adulthood. This is because of years and years of slow erosion and constant acidic build up. This condition is reversed by eating more alkaline foods until the problem is healed. The ratio should be 80% raw alkaline producing and 20% acidic producing cooked foods.

Follow Daily Meal Planner: Add flax seed oil, olive oil, slippery elm

Heal and Prevent Depression, Fatigue and Migraines

Sugar not only causes suppression of the immune system, but it also throws all of the body hormone producing organs out of whack. Sugar and lack of natural minerals in their proper balance is the number one cause of depression. Sugar contributes to over 130 diseases and it insidiously weakens the entire body over time. Sugar is highly acidic and addictive. Sugar causes your food to spoil in your intestines and is a false source of energy that tricks the body. It is highly addictive and habit forming just like heroin. Sugar stresses out the organs in the body bringing on constant fatigue. Sugar is a great contributor to migraines, because it shuts off oxygen to the brain. The best thing that anyone can do is to completely remove all sugar and products containing sugar from their diet. If I taste just the slightest amount of sugar, I will immediately start feeling depressed and sluggish. Sugar immediately poisons the blood because it lacks fiber and other nutrients that healthy food contains. It immediately shuts off oxygen supply to the cells, thus shutting down the body's systems. This is why if you are suffering any type of degenerative disease like cancer, obesity, heart disease, hypertension, and diabetes it is imperative that you avoid all refined sugars and products that contain sugar. A reduction in sugar greatly improves emotional stability. Add Celtic Sea Salt to your diet to help regulate hormone imbalances and curb sugar cravings.

Follow Daily Meal Planner: Use stevia, honey, 100% maple syrup

Heal and Prevent Rheumatoid Arthritis

Arthritis comes in many different forms as a result of acid build up in the joints and wrist. The body will take selenium from the joints in order to neutralize this acid build up. Selenium helps to keep the joints from drying out. Over time, this constant depletion of selenium causes the joints to lose their elasticity and become weak and brittle. This results in inflammation between the joints which leads to what we call arthritis. If this acidic condition is not corrected it can get worse and even become crippling.

Follow Daily Meal Planner:

Herbs: Boswellia, Bromelain, Tumeric, Cat's claw, Ginger, Cayenne

Heal and Prevent Colds and Flus

Colds and flus are simply bacterial infections that are able to overtake the body when the body's immune system is not properly functioning. Sugar is the number one suppressor of the body's immune system. One teaspoon of sugar will shut the immune system down for up to 12 hours. Because of the average American diet, 99.9% of the general population never has full use of their immune systems their entire lives. When your immune system is in proper working order, the body will respond to the symptom and arrest the virus before it can manifest into an infectious disease. I have found this to be true in myself and in others. I don't get colds or the flu, just the symptoms. The key to preventing these kinds of illnesses is to keep your immune system healthy. The next time you feel a cold coming on, stop all intake of sugar from all sources. Drink an 8-ounce glass of water mixed with ½ fresh squeezed lemon, 1/4 teaspoon of Celtic Sea Salt sweetened with stevia. Drink this once every four hours. In between, drink lemon and water. It is imperative that during this time you avoid all refined sugar and foods that contain sugar in them. The symptoms should clear up within a day or two. If you want to keep your immune system at full operating level, raw organic garlic should be consumed daily. Consume organic raw garlic for four weeks as this will restore your immune system.

Herbs: Cat's claw, Echinacea, Elderberry, Ginger, Garlic, Hyssop

Heal and Prevent Gout

This condition is a direct result of an over-consumption of meat products. Today animals and fish are raised strictly for com-mercial purposes. They are injected with antibiotics just to keep them alive until they reach the slaughter houses and processing plants. The meat of these commercial animals are full of growth hormones and synthetically processed foods. These foods are mixed together with other dead animals that were too diseased to make it to slaughter. The animals never get to exercise because they are stuck in cages, thus the toxins they produce stay in them their entire lifetime. Humans simply consume too much of this highly toxic junk and one of the damaging by-products created is uric acid. This acid settles in the joints, espe-cially those of the big toe, which can be very painful. The best way to prevent this condition is to eat meat once or twice a month. Al-ways boil your chicken and turkey before you eat it. And try to eat animals and fish that are non-farm raised.

Follow Daily Meal Planner: Add grapefruit seed extract, flax seed oil
Herbs: Bilberry, celery seed, Devil's claw, Quercetin, Sarsaparilla

Heal and Prevent Elevated Cholesterol

The problem with the average American diet is that we eat too many animal and dairy products, thus overloading the blood with excess cholesterol. Seafood and ham are especially high in cholesterol and is probably why God commanded that they not be eaten, to protect mankind. Turkey and chicken also contain elevated levels of cholesterol and should be eaten sparingly. Meat in moderation does not cause any problems and is okay as long as it is lean and you trim off the fat. If you must have meat, it should only be eaten once a week or every other week. You can get plenty of protein from plant, grains, beans, yeast, seeds, and nut sources. Apes in the wild who don't eat meat are healthier than we are. Watch your intake of processed dairy products and eat more naturally small scaled fish instead. Sugar also causes the body to produce more cholesterol, so watch or completely avoid refined sugar.

Follow Daily Meal Planner:
Herbs: Artichoke leaf, Garlic, Ginseng, Hawthorn, Spirulina, Shiitake

Heal and Prevent Osteoporosis

This disease causes bones to degenerate and decrease in mass. It affects millions of men and women worldwide. In America alone, more than 10 million people are currently struggling with osteoporosis. Fifty percent of women and 12% of men will be affected by osteoporosis in their lifetime. To heal this condition, one must eat foods rich in all natural minerals available in Celtic Sea Salt. It is also important to avoid foods, beverages, and man-made mineral supplements that leach minerals from the bones and cause them to lose their density. Hydration is vitally important as the bones are comprised of up to 35% water. Lack of water and certain bone hardening minerals is the greatest cause of this disease. Sugar is also a contributing factor as it weakens the entire skeletal structure of the body, because it leaches minerals from the marrow of the bones. In elderly people, one of the greatest life threatening risks is bone fractures due to accidental falls. The important thing to remember is the fact that you are not born with this condition, so it can be reversed though it may take some time.

Follow Daily Meal Planner: Add sunflower seeds and flax seed oil.
Herbs: Alfalfa, Feverfew, Hawthorn, Por huesos.

Heal and Prevent Obesity

This problem is simply an overexposure to slow burning, highly acidic foods and lack of aerobic activity. Overingestion of carbohydrates and fats, without enough exercise to burn them as fuel, causes our bodies to store them as fatty acids. This prevents the cellular engines from burning on all cylinders, reducing out metabolic rate. So with a combination of lack of exercise, which reduces oxygen, toxic acidic residues builds around the cells. Infiltration of morbid microforms in and around the cell and a reduction of peak performance energy burning from the mitochondria engines, allows obesity to set in. With the obesity problem in this country, what exactly does this excess weight consist of? The answer is fatty acids. However, the body does not dispose of unburned food. This unburned food or fatty acids are stored in fat cells until they can be burned at a later time through some form of aerobics. To a point, it is a reservoir to be burned later, but if later never comes then we keep adding to the fatty acid reservoir.

Acid coagulates blood and there is not much blood flow around fat. Usually the capillaries around the acid accumulation are clogged up. These fatty acids generally form under the skin, especially around the waistline for men and around hips, thighs and breasts for women. When you compare the face of an old woman with a young woman, you can see the difference in the build up of fat in the face of the older woman due to lack of blood flow, therefore losing elasticity. This build up of fat in the face takes place gradually over time. True understanding of the process of aging and obesity will give you the incentive to drink alkaline beverages and eat alkaline foods that burn fast. Whatever it takes to help your body dispose of acidic waste slowly and steadily should be implemented.
Herbs: Aloe vera, Astragalus, Ephedra, Mate, Wild angelica

Heal and Prevent Allergies

Allergies are an inflamation appearing as allergy symptoms which are a result of the body dealing wit acidic toxic build up. Foods like dairy products, non-organic eggs, and processed wheat products greatly complicate allergic reactions. Fresh-squeezed lemon juice and lots of dark green leafy vegetables will reduce or totally eliminate tearing eyes, runny nose, sinus swelling, and skin reactions. The acidic waste from yeast and fungus are also contributing factors and should be eliminated with thorough internal cleansing. When the immune system is compromised and toxic acids build up in the body, you will have to deal with sinus problems.

Follow Daily Meal Planner: Add fresh lemon juice and spinach.

Herbs: Agrimony, Chamomile, Ginger, Peppermint, Calendula

Heal and Prevent Cysts and Tumors (benign)

These two conditions normally are not life threatening, but can cause discomfort and disfiguring. To prevent cysts, it is important that you remove all dairy from your diet with the exception of raw organic yogurt and certain types of organic cheeses. Both tumors and cysts are a result of over-acidification in the blood which the body collects and pushes out of the way. This can easily be reversed and prevented by eating a much more alkaline diet and using a blood purifier like grapefruit seed extract.

Follow Daily Meal Planner: Add grapefruit seed extract.

Heal and Prevent Inflammation

This condition is a lot more common than generally thought. Over-acidification for extended periods of time is the major culprit behind this disease. In the same way that battery acid can cause severe burns upon contact with the skin, high acidification in the blood exposes the cells to the same type of condition. When the skin is exposed to acid, it burns and swells. This swelling is a form of inflammation. A highly acidic diet causes the same type of burning and swelling to our cells. Over an extended period of time, this eventually leads to inflammation which settles in the weakest links of the body, i.e. joints and organs. To prevent and totally heal this condition, change to a 70% raw and 30% cooked diet.

Follow Daily Meal Planner: Add grapefruit seed extract, grapefruits.

Heal and Prevent Autoimmune Disease

This condition causes the body's immune system to attack itself

by mistake. Autoimmune disease affects various areas of the body like the joints, nerves, muscles, endocrine system, and digestive system. The disease is classified into five classes: lupus, Grave's disease, multiple sclerosis, rheumatoid arthritis, and underactive thyroid. These five categories include over 40 common ailments that adversely affect women more than men. This condition is directly linked to poor nutrition and assimilation. You see, it really doesn't matter what you eat if the end result does not meet the needs of your cells. If your cells are unhealthy and starved, the rest of your body will manifest this internal condition. You must eat more living raw foods, exercise, and get plenty of rest. This condition and the other 40 diseases associated with it can be healed and prevented through proper nutritional habits. It is also important to eat foods that enhance the immune system and avoid immune compromising substances.
Follow Daily Meal Planner. Garlic, dark greens, citrus fruits

Heal and Prevent Bowel Disease

Almost 600,000 Americans suffer with this condition which causes abdominal cramps and pain, diarrhea, weight loss and bleeding from the intestines. While the medical community has not found the cause for this ailment, in my opinion, it is directly related to an over-acidic diet. Acids are very caustic substances which can burn very quickly or slowly depending on the type of acid. Since the body produces acid naturally, adding more can cause a whole host of problems. This is similar to cholesterol in animal products that cause the body to produce higher, unhealthy levels of cholesterol. A quick, easy, and inexpensive way to correct this condition is to simply change over to a 90% raw and 10% cooked diet. Eat a lot of fresh, dark green leafy vegetables and fruits. Avoid coffee, soda, and drink plenty of water. Try to make your own fruit juice and avoid drinking commercially processed fruit drinks.
Follow Daily Meal Planner: Add slippery elm, ground flax seed.
Herbs: Alfalfa, lemon balm, Peppermint, Psyllium seed, Rosemary

Heal and Prevent Anemia

This condition is brought about by prescription medications and poor nutritional habits. The body loses it ability to produce red blood cells within the marrow of the bones. Or the body turns on itself and mistakenly destroys red blood cells. This condition is known as auto-immune hemolytic anemia. Poor dietary iron intake or excessive bleeding can also contribute to this condition. There are many forms of anemia, with the most common forms being corrected through proper nutrition. It is best to use an all-natural approach to correct this problem versus toxic medication that can further exacerbate this condition.

Follow Daily Meal Planner: Spinach, kale, greens, figs, nuts, seeds, sesame seeds, and small scaled fish.

Herbs: Dandelion, Stinging nettle

Heal and Prevent Kidney Failure

The kidneys are responsible for flushing waste out of the body. They act as a filter for the blood stream and are extremely overtaxed when the blood has too much acidic waste and heavy metals. This acid eats away at the kidneys leading to kidney failure over time. A salt-free diet is deadly to the kidneys, because the kidneys have to work extra hard to remove excess minerals from the blood. Table salt, dairy products, and cooked meats produce phosphoric and uric acid combined with calcium and magnesium that gradually build up into stones. These stones are very painful in the kidneys and bladder. With an alkaline diet, internal cleansing, and Celtic Sea Salt, these stones will dissolve from within. Diabetic and high blood pressure medcations greatly contribute to kidney failure. One must do all that they can to completely discontinue the use of medications as soon as possible. The side affects from these medications far outweigh their benefits over an extended period of time. As soon as your kidneys are healed, consult with your physician about cutting back on medica-tions. You should reach the point where medications are no longer needed.

Follow Daily Meal Planner. Ginseng, grape seed extract.

Herbs: Abuta, Bupleurum, Dandelion root, Marshmallow root

Heal and Prevent MS

Again, we have another autoimmune disease that causes the body to attack itself. This sinister diseases normally shows up at around the age of 30 and can lead to permanent disability and eventually premature death. This condition causes the immune system to attack nerve fibers and interferes with electrical impulses. It causes various symptoms like bladder and bowel dysfunction and vision problems. One's nutritional history will have a great impact on the severity of this disease. This disease is totally reversible and must be aggressively attacked with immune-boosting foods, exercise, plenty of water and detoxing.

Follow Daily Meal Planner. Add super green foods, whole foods, vegetable-based supplements, garlic, flaxseed oil.

Herbs: Alfalfa, Ginkgo, Soy Lecithin

Heal and Prevent PMS Complications

There is not an exact known cause for this condition, but it is believed lifestyle habits play a major role. One thing that is known, when woman goes through PMS, she loses a lot of vital trace minerals, minerals and hormones. It is important that women replace these minerals on a daily basis. These minerals will help to regulate the production of hormones and counter the symptoms of hormonal imbalances. Some of the symptoms associated with PMS are headaches, swelling of ankles, backache, abdominal cramps, abdominal pain, muscle spasms, breast tenderness, weight gain, acne, nausea, bloating, constipation, and diarrhea. Other symptoms include, anxiety, confusion, forgetfulness, depression, and fatigue. Some of the lifestyles changes often recommended for the treatment of PMS may actually be useful in preventing symptoms from developing or getting worse. Regular exercise and a balanced diet that include an increased intake of whole grains, vegetables, fruit, and decreased or no sugar, alcohol, and caffeine may prove beneficial. All natural Celtic Sea Salt is important along with plenty of distilled water. All sugar and artificial sweeteners should be avoided and replaced with stevia, maple syrup, and honey. The body may have different sleep requirements at different times during a woman's menstrual cycle, so it is important to get adequate rest.

Heal and Prevent Liver Disease (NASH)

The liver is one of the most vital organs in the body next to the heart and brain. It is responsible for cleansing the blood, regulating the productions of certain hormones, burning excess fat, and distributing fat evenly throughout the body. The liver is a very sensitive organ and is often damaged by heavy metals, acidic build up, toxins, prescription medications, and trans-fats. When the liver is not collecting fat from the blood and sending it out of the body through the gut, it is dangerously storing fat and eventually becomes just a bag of fat. When this occurs, the liver no longer functions and fat starts to collect between the waist-line and lower chest. People with this condition have a very difficult time losing weight, and often have problems with hormonal imbalances. With the extended presence of toxic waste forming in the blood, the body signals that death is occurring. So certain cells respond by transforming themselves for the task of decomposing the body. This is where the majority of degenerative diseases start to set in. Fortunately, this condition is reversible and within four months, you can have a completely new liver.

Follow Daily Meal Planner. Add liver detox, milk thistle.

Herbs: Astragalus, Cinnamon, Lentinan, Scutellaria, goldenseal

Heal and Prevent Acid Reflux

Your stomach is full of acids that are just as strong as battery acid. The stomach can handle these acids, but your esophagus can't. So through improper food combinations and highly acidic foods, acid backs up into the esophagus causing burning. This occurs when the lower sphincter valve separating the stomach and esophagus does not properly close during digestion, allowing stomach acids to escape. If not treated, this disease can destroy the inner lining of the esophagus, but it is reversible through a mineral-rich diet using Celtic Sea Salt and proper food combinations. Herbs like Slippery Elm and olive oil can be used to soothe and coat your esophagus. Olive oil will reduce the intensity of the acid and add alkalinity to your diet. A diet rich in fruits, essential fatty oils, flax seeds, nuts, and vegetables are very beneficial to alleviating this condition. Avoid sugary drinks with your meals as this only adds more acid to the stomach. Drink distilled water, all natural lemonade, and herbal teas sweetened with stevia or honey.

Heal and Prevent Poor Circulation Diseases

Lately, more and more television commercials are advertising drugs to treat circulation diseases like peripheral artery disease. This disease involves arteries and veins outside of the heart and brain. It involves a narrowing of vessels that carry blood to the stomach, legs, arms, and liver. This disease is similar to coronary heart disease where fatty deposits builds up in the inner linings of the artery walls. This restricts blood circulation causing fatigue and cramping of the legs and buttocks during activity. This condition is directly related to nutritional habits and smoking. It is easily reversed through an all-natural diet of fruits, vegetables, and certain cooked meats like chicken, and poultry. This ailment can be debilitating if not properly treated aggressively in a timely fashion. Oxygen-depleting, highly acidic foods greatly complicate this condition along with the consumption of refined sugar, lunch-meat and hot dogs, sausages, and hydrogenated products. Change to 95% raw and 5% cooked meals until the condition reverses itself. Upon recovery, limit or restrict consumption of processed meats.

Follow Daily Meal Planner: Liver detox, ginseng, asparagus.

Herbs: Aconite, Asparagus root, Hawthorn, Motherwort, Astragalus

Heal and Prevent Fungal Infections

The body normally hosts a variety of microorganisms including fungi. Some of these are useful to the body. Others may multiply rapidly and form infections. Fungi can live on the dead tissues of the hair, nails, and outer skin layers. Types of fungal infections are athlete's foot, jock itch, ringworm, tinea capitis, yeast infections, finger and toe nail infection, oral thrush, cutaneous candida, and some rashes. Fungal nail infections may be difficult to treat and may recur often. Toenails are affected more often than fingernails. Avoiding tight fitting shoes and changing socks frequently is the first place to start. Whenever possible, wear sandals or open-toed shoes. A parasitic cleanse is very effective as well as drinking grapefruit seed extract daily. Garlic is also effective in controlling the overgrowth of fungus, unhealthy yeast, and parasites.

Herbs: Barberry, Coix, Echinacea, Pau d'arco, walnut leaf, Scutellaria

Heal and Prevent Menopause

Women are born with roughly one to three million eggs, which are gradually lost throughout their lifetime. The eggs are stored in the ovaries where estrogen and progesterone are stored, which regulate menstruation and ovulation. Menopause occurs when the ovaries are totally depleted of eggs and no amount of stimulation from the regulating hormones can force them to work. By the time a girl reaches the age of 12-14, she has an average of 400,000 eggs. When starting menopause, a woman only has 10,000 eggs left. At the age of 45 and 55, a woman goes through menopause as a normal part of life. This condition can come on earlier, but such cases are premature as a result of damaged ovaries or some type of surgical procedure. A large number of eggs die off and others are lost through menstruation every month. Early symptoms include abnormal vaginal bleeding, hot flashes, and mood changes. Late symptoms include vaginal dryness and irritation. Exercise, natural mineral replacement through properly salted foods, flaxseed oil, and avoidance of refined sugar and artificial sweeteners. This approach is very effective in beating the odds of suffering with menopause.

Herbs: Aloe, Black cohosh, Calendula, Dong quai, Ginseng, Vitex

Heal and Prevent Poor Vision

This condition affects one in three persons living in this country. There are many contributing factors, but in my opinion, they all come right back to refined sugar or artificial sweeteners, parasitic infestation, and hydrogenated oils. Lack of exercise and a lifestyle of mainly cooked foods can both be contributing factors. Some of the smallest veins and blood vessels are located in the eyes. These can easily become clogged, and the muscles in the eyes have to strain to focus, which eventually causes weakness and poor vision. To prevent and reverse this condition, a lifestyle change is necessary. Avoiding sugar completely will be the greatest benefit and have lasting affects. Exercise will keep the veins and arteries in a youthful condition. Celtic Sea Salt will flush the arteries and remove plaque and film from the eyes.

Follow Daily Meal Planner. Total body detox, ginseng, spinach

Heal and Prevent Parasitic Infestation

Everyone has parasites and under normal conditions, they don't cause any problems. However, when the immune system is compromised mainly through poor nutritional habits, these parasites can grow into an infestation and start causing all types of medical problems. Sugar causes your meals to spoil in your stomach which leads to fermentation. This type of environment allows the parasites to thrive unchecked. If not treated, they can attack your organs and cause all types of medical complications. Many doctors don't treat this condition, because they are not trained thoroughly regarding this very common problem. There are several ways to treat this condition and bring it under control. A parasitic cleansing should be done at least once a year. There are several types of cleansing products you can buy in your local health food store. Garlic, cilantro, pumpkin seeds, and black walnut husk are foods you can add to your diet that greatly inhibit the growth of parasites. Celtic Sea Salt is effective in that it works as an antiseptic, which slows the growth of micro organisms.
Herbs: Agrimony, Barberry, Black walnut, Echinacea, Garlic, Lpecac

Heal and Prevent Impotency

Erectile dysfunction is the inability to obtain or maintain an erection. It is not a disease, but a symptom of an underlying problem, the most common being diabetes. Diabetes can cause changes in blood flow through narrowing of the arteries or damaged nerve endings in the penis. Nutritional habits and smoking are other contributing factors causing arterial blockages, reducing blood flow necessary to maintain an erection. Roughly 30 million men in the United states suffer with this condition and it is up to 95% treatable. The most common medication used to treat this disorder is Viagra, but not without side affects like headaches, facial flushing, upset stomach, backache, and blindness. With all of the adverse side affects, I suggest trying an all-natural approach. There are some very powerful herbal remedies you can use for example. Ginseng Complex, Maui Parana, and organic garlic are a very powerful and potent combination. All improve circulation to every area of the body and even strengthens arteries, something Viagra can't do. Simply follow the directions and only use if you have regular sexual intimacy with your spouse.

Herbs: Ashwaganda, Damiana, Ginseng, Morinda, Muira puama

Heal and Prevent Peripheral Artery Disease

This disease is extremely dangerous and affects 12 to 15 million people annually. It is often mis-diagnosed and can lead to a sudden heart attack and premature death. Diabetics and smokers are highly susceptible to this diseases. This condition is caused by poor circulation and hardening of the arteries with symptoms not developing until the artery is nearly 60% defective. The body will grow new arteries to channel blood flow around the defective area, and this explains why one doesn't develop any symptoms until it's too late. When a piece of damaged artery or clot breaks away from the lining of the artery, or the artery is completely blocked, the organ supplied by that artery will eventually die. This can lead to gangrene and eventually amputation. It is imperative that immediate measures are taken to reverse this disease as it will only worsen. Lifestyle changes and heavy detoxing along with 10 to12 glasses of distilled water per day. The good news is the disease is totally reversible if handled in a timely fashion. Avoid all processed meats, especially hot dogs and sausage meats. Garlic, olive oil, and flaxseed oil should be consumed daily until condition clears up.

Follow Daily Meal Planner: Liver detox, ginseng, organic broccoli. Add diced garlic placed into a gel cap.

Heal and Prevent Acne

This is a common condition that mostly affects adolescents, but can carry over into adulthood. It is directly related to nutritional habits, dehydration, and lack of exercise. The body is severely acidic, and skin eruptions like acne, is the body's way of pushing these toxins out. It is very easy to treat and normally will clear up within a few weeks after cleansing and a thorough detox. The vast majority of people who suffer with this disease are not born with it, which means it can only develop as a result of what we have exposed ourselves to. Processed foods, junk food, soft drinks, and high amounts of refined sodium are very toxic. These toxins build up over time and eventually lead to acne and other skin eruptions.

Follow Daily Meal Planner: Liver detox, ginseng, asparagus.

Herbs: Walnut leaf, Milk thistle, Saw palmetto, Tea tree oil, Giggul

Heal and Prevent Mineral Deficiencies

Believe it or not, mineral deficiencies are a major culprit behind a vast majority of the common ailments in this country, especially mental and physiological disorders. Most of the food harvested in this country comes from mineral-depleted soils. If the soil is void of minerals, then the food will be in the same condition. Also the heavy use of commercial fertilizers causes our fruits and vegetables to absorb high levels of unbalanced minerals. Fortified minerals are not recognized by the body and are in unnaturally high concentrations when added back to our foods. Every function of the body requires minerals, especially digestion. Without minerals, proper digestion and assimilation is all but impossible. Intravenous feeding is a solution of minerals used to save lives in emergency rooms all around the country. I can't stress the importance of having the proper balance of minerals in your daily diet. One must be very careful when purchasing commercially-processed minerals. Some minerals, like trace minerals, are needed in very minute quantities. An overabundance of minerals can cause just as many health problems as being mineral deficient. The best way to ensure that you get all of your minerals is to daily sprinkle Celtic Sea Salt on all of your foods. That's right, on everything you eat. It is best to use after cooking by allowing the moisture in your food to interact with the salt before eating. Simply sprinkle the salt on your food and allow it to stand for two or three minutes. Remember, table salt only contains two minerals, sodium and chlorine, in unhealthy amounts. It also has chemicals that prevent digestion by blocking the formation of stomach acids. Throw out the table salt and use real, naturally-balanced sea salt from now on.

Heal and Prevent Hyperactivity

In my opinion, this condition results from too many artificial sweeteners and food colorings. Today, the foods we consume are artificial and no longer grazed but fed pelletized animal feed. Our food

supply is totally deficient of nutrients and minerals. The brain is very complex and requires a vast array of vitamins, amino acids, minerals, and nutrients, to produce neurotransmitters. Without proper production of these chemicals, the brain cannot communicate. Also, it is well known that fluorescent lighting can have the same adverse affects as a mineral deficiency. In laboratory tests, male rats must be removed before the female gives birth to avoid cannibalism. This only occurs under fluorescent lighting. With full spectrum lighting that resemble the wave lengths of natural sunlight, the male rat will actually nurture the new-born. We are born drinking artificial milk and grow up eating artificial foods. However, God did not create us with artificial blood, cells, or organs. Refined sugar and artificial sweeteners are poisonous and foreign to the human body. The body's natural response is to try and force these toxins out. Hyperactivity is an attempt of the body in trying to throw off these poisons as quickly as possible. Before the 1950s, food coloring was accomplished by using plant extracts. These new petroleum-based colorings were cheaper and also preserved foods. The brain cannot deal with the large number of food colorings circulating in the blood. The only way to heal and prevent this condition is to return to a diet of 80% raw and 20% cooked foods. Add Celtic Sea Salt, Flax seed oil, and ginseng.
Herbs: Avena, Chamomile, Ginkgo, Hawthorn, Lobelia, Scutellaria

Heal and Prevent Indigestion

This condition is caused by a number of contributing factors to include smoking and bacterial infestation like Helicobacter pylori. Prescription drugs, aspirin, and anti-inflammatory medications can irritate the situation. If not treated, it can eventually lead to cancer in some people. Foods eaten in the wrong combinations or going long periods without food can cause a build up of stomach acids. A heavy meal can also exacerbate this condition along with alcohol and smoking. Eating smaller meals more frequently can ease the problem. Nutritional lifestyle changes will totally reverse this acidic disease.
Follow Daily Meal Planner. Water, olive oil, ground flax seed.
Herbs: Chen-pi, Fennel seed, Ginger, Peppermint

Heal and Prevent Alcoholism and Drug Addiction

Refined white sugar and white salt are great contributors to both problems. The salt is a major culprit, because it lacks the minerals needed by the brain to function properly, making it more difficult to make sound decisions. Refined sugar actually cuts off oxygen to the brain, and also poisons every cell in the body. With your body constantly in a condition of lack, trying to survive and function properly at the same time can lead to an overload of the system, causing undue stress and poor decision making. Remember, drug and alcohol addictions are not diseases, they are choices one makes. A person would have to decide if their health is more important than the drugs and alcohol. When everything is functioning properly, making that decision becomes easier.

There are millions of drug users in this country and for many of them, all it took was one time to become a regular user. The main reason people use drugs is because they induce a feeling of happiness. No one likes pain, mental or physical. Alcohol has the same type of affect, and if not controlled, can lead to sclerosis of the liver. Alcohol and drugs negatively impact earnings because of reduced labor productivity. A diet high in refined sugar and artificial sweeteners, like high fructose corn syrup, can lead to alcohol dependancy. High fructose corn syrup interferes with many hormonal functions and communication processes between the brain and organs like the pancreas. A proper diet can greatly reduce the dependancy and need for alcohol and drugs.

Follow Daily Meal Planner. Liver detox, avoid artificial sweeteners.
Herbs: Kudzu, Milk thistle, Reishi, Soy lecithin

Heal and Prevent Gallstones

This condition hospitalizes some 800,000 people annually, making it the most costly digestive disease in the United States. More than 20 million people suffer with this condition, which strikes women more often than men. It is believed that treating this disorder costs over $5 billion annually. People who are overweight and past the age of 30 are typical patients; however, younger people are starting to develop gallstones. The function of the bladder is to store bile produced by the liver, and to aid in digestion and absorption of fats. Gallstones compose a solid formation of cholesterol and bile salts. Today, the average diet is loaded with cholesterol which causes the liver to produce bile that is overly saturated with cholesterol, which then crystallizes and forms stones. Bile acids and lecithin in low amounts can also lead to stones. This condition is directly related to poor nutritional habits and dehydration. Changing to an 85% raw and 15% cooked diet will help reverse this problem. Use whole Celtic Sea Salt and drink plenty of water. The symptoms from this disease can be very misleading and are often mis-diagnosed.

Follow Daily Meal Planner: Liver detox; natural juicing; baked or broiled fish; avoid artificial sweeteners.

Herbs: Peppermint, Prickly ash, Alfalfa, Boldo, Milk thistle, Tumeric

Heal and Prevent Hemorrhoids

This condition is the result of too much pressure on the veins of the anus. It can be as a result of constipation or straining to pass hard stools. It can also be caused by excessive rubbing and cleaning around the rectum area. Most people lack insoluble fiber in their diets, and are dehydrated most of the time. These two factors can make stools hard and difficult to pass. Some people who suffer with hemorrhoids can develop certain types of cancers. Chronic diarrhea, aging, pregnancy, frequent use of laxatives, enemas, and heredity can play a role also. A change in nutritional habits can greatly reverse this condition. Olive oil, flax seed oil, ground flax seed, and water should be consumed immediately. Drink at least six to eight glasses of water daily and eat more water soluble foods.

Herbs: Aloe, Calendula, St. John's Wort, Dandelion, Horse tail

Heal and Prevent Sugar Addiction

Roughly 95% of all people living in this country are addicted to refined sugar and artificial sweeteners. Sugar is responsible for a host of degenerative diseases. One of the main reasons for this addiction is the absence of minerals needed for proper digestion. Without these minerals to counter and balance out the body, sugar cravings will occur as a result. It is amazing to hear people tell me about how they kicked the sugar habit by simply adding Celtic Sea Salt to their diet daily. Minerals are needed to properly break down food for digestion. The food we eat is turned into sugar to be used as energy for the body. In the absence of these sugars, the body will crave out other sources of sugar to compensate. Once this imbalance is overcome, which takes about three to four months, the desire and cravings for sugar will slowly start diminishing. Add more natural proteins to your diet, like nuts and beans, this will help satisfy your sweet tooth. **Follow Daily Meal Planner**. Add fresh fruits, ground flax seed

Heal and Prevent Varicose Veins

This condition affects up to 60% of all women and men in this country; however, women suffer more. Arteries carry blood throughout the body and veins carry blood back to the heart. If the veins become weak, blood will back up into the vein becoming congested and clogged. This will cause the veins to enlarge abnormally resulting in varicose or spider veins. They appear in the legs most often, because this area has to work harder to send blood back to the heart due to gravity. In my opinion, this condition is caused by sugar and artificial sweeteners, a lack of real sea salt, and hydrogenated oils. Garlic, exercise, olive oil, and naturally-mineralized salt can help greatly in reversing this unsightly condition.
Herbs: Bromelain, Butchers broom, Cayenne, Hawthorn, Gotu kola

Heal and Prevent Eczema

This condition is a direct result of over acidity in the blood. When a diet full of sugar and artificial sweeteners is added, this condition worsens drastically. It can be inherited and become very irritating and painful if not managed properly. Fortunately, this condition can be reversed with a change in nutritional habits. First, you'll need to do a total body detox and daily cleansing. Avoid all sodas and drinks sweetened with sugar, corn syrup, or any other artificial sweetener. Distilled water is one of the cheapest and most effective ways to jump start the reversal process. Natural juicing should be implemented along with all-natural lemonade sweetened with stevia or maple syrup. A diet consisting of 85% raw and 15% cooked foods should be consumed daily until the condition clears up. Fried foods, junk foods, and certain types of lotions should also be avoided. A combination of olive oil and grapefruit seed extract can be used in place of lotions. Add 1/8 teaspoon of Celtic Sea Salt to your drinking water at least once a day. Once this condition is reversed, carefully monitor your nutritional habits to prevent acidic build up in the blood. **Follow Daily Meal Planner**. Add fresh fruits, flax seed oil, greens. **Herbs**: Aloe, Avena, Chamomile, Rosemary, Turmeric, Walnut leaf

Heal and Prevent Learning Disorders

It would be difficult to learn properly if you didn't have the required curriculum. In the same manner, without the balance of minerals and fats needed for proper brain function, one will have a difficult time learning. Because everyone's body chemistry is so different, some people suffer more severely with this imbalance than others. Also, heavy metal poisoning can make learning very difficult. We are exposed to these metals from a myriad of sources, environmental and domestic. There are metal detox cleansers available, along with reduced sugar intake that can make a major difference. Adding Celtic Sea Salt will bring an overall balance to the entire body, and help reduce stress, making it easier to focus and retain information. Refined and artificial sweeteners to include sugar and Splenda™ are toxic, and cause the body to spend more energy on survival than any other function. This information is just a general overview of certain conditions that can make learning difficult. You can do your own research to further uncover other areas that contribute to this problem. For the most part, our diets are deficient in minerals and EFAs that are vitally needed for proper brain function. For almost the past 60 years, these two important nutrients have been missing from the American landscape.
Follow Daily Meal Planner: Celtic Sea Salt, Flax seed oil, and water

Heal and Prevent Emotional Instability

The human body is an amazing piece of work and can function under the most impossible situations. If what we consume causes us to become stressed inwardly, then we will display physical manifestation. Refined sugar is definitely associated with emotional and hormonal imbalances, and depletes the body of oxygen. It also leaches vital minerals and trace minerals that are needed for the body to function properly. In psychiatric wards and discipline boot camps, sugar intake is greatly reduced to help calm aggressive individuals. If you are suffering with any type of emotional imbalances, immediately remove all refined sugar and artificial sweeteners, commercial seasonings, table salt, and processed foods from your diet. Eat whole foods that are unprocessed and are as fresh as possible. Drink plenty of distilled water, add Celtic Sea salt to all meals and take flax seed oil daily.

Follow Daily Meal Planner: Add fresh fruits, ground flaxseed, greens.
Herbs: Coptis, Echinacea, slippery elm, bark, Red clover, Dong Quai

Heal and Prevent Boils

Boils are skin eruptions that can appear suddenly and be very painful. It is usually caused by staphylococcal bacteria, and most always with a head that will normally burst. This condition will result when the blood is polluted and in need of purification. The best way to treat this condition is to use grapefruit seed extract, which is a blood purifier. Healthier nutritional habits can greatly reduce the occurrence of this condition. Boiling meats before cooking removes a lot of the impurities in the meat that defile the blood. Remember, the life of the flesh is in the blood. **Remember, God has placed before you life and death, sickness and disease, so choose life, that you and your seed may live.**

C H A P T E R   16

Importance of Vitamins and Minerals

"I have set before you life and death, blessing and cursing: therefore choose life, that both thou and thy seed may live:" (Deuteronomy 30:19)

Many people take vitamins and supplements to ensure that they are properly meeting all of their nutritional needs. With the poor quality of our soils today, bio-genetic tampering, scientific manipulation and over processing of the food supply, a person has every reason to be concerned. However the question still remains, are these supplements really all they're cracked up to be? After all, they have been around for a long time, yet degenerative diseases continue to reach historical levels. This is an excellent question whose answer is straight forward. Synthetic vitamins are not recognized by nor are they assimilated in the body. Again, I point to the fact that you were not made out of synthetic material, but real living organic matter. Therefore, your source of vitamins and minerals must be from the same source. The body does not produce vitamins in sufficient enough amounts to meet all of our nutritional needs, so they must be obtained through our diets.

The problem is our food supply is vitamin deficient because of contaminated soils and industrial processing. Also, exposure to light will degrade and destroy a lot of vitamins. Most vitamins are light and heat sensitive. This is why cooking at high temperatures is so unhealthy, because it totally destroys all of the vital nutrients contained in the food. Vitamins are called essential nutrients and are needed by the body to heal, protect, and prevent disease. Vitamins protect our hearts from damage and protect us against cancer. Recent research evidence also suggests that vitamin C and E combined in high doses helps reduce our risk of developing Alzheimer's disease.

Since it is hard to obtain a balanced diet from the foods we consume today, I do recommend taking a vitamin supplement, but not just any kind of supplement. Remember, the body must stay balanced in order to properly function. Taking vitamins and minerals in high dosages is absolutely never recommended. It's better that you take smaller dosages and let your body heal itself over time than to take more than the body can handle at one time and cause severe damage.

Whole food supplements, produced under very strict guidelines to ensure the highest product quality, are the best. They may be a little more expensive, because they are vegetable based and organic, but they are really the only way to go if you are going to take supplements. Otherwise, you are simply wasting your money as again, the human body will not assimilate synthetic supplements. A lot of these supplements through over exposure can actually cause more damage than good. I wouldn't recommend taking synthetic mineral supplements under any circumstance. Overexposure to minerals and certain trace minerals can be fatal. Your minerals and trace minerals should only come from properly balanced, unrefined, moist, light gray Celtic Sea Salt. This should be sprinkled over all of your foods in moderation, and always drink plenty of water to maximize the effectiveness of the minerals inside the body.

Vitamin A: Helps regulate the immune system, which helps prevent and combat infections by producing white blood cells that destroy harmful bacteria and viruses and help lymphocytes (a type of white blood cell that help us fight infections) function more vigorously. Vitamin A also plays a significant role in vision, bone growth, reproduction, cell division and cell differentiation. It helps to maintain the membranous linings of the eyes and the respiratory, urinary, and intestinal tracts. Those linings protect the organs from being invaded by bacteria and viruses. Vitamin A in its beta-carotene form neutralizes free radicals through its antioxidant properties. May also protect against cancer of the lung, breast, bladder, prostate and digestive tract. It inhibits abnormal cell growth, strengthens the immune system, and aids and fortifies cellular functions.

Vitamin C: Is essential for the manufacturing of collagen and necessary for tissue repair. It is needed for metabolism of phenylalanine, tyrosine, folic acid, iron. Vitamin C is also vital for healthy immune and nervous systems because it strengthens blood vessels, as it is an anti-oxidant that participates in oxidation-reduction reactions.

Health Benefits: Vitamin C is one of the most crucial vitamins in your body and in fact, plays a large role in hundreds of the body's functions. The most plentiful tissue in the body is collagen, which is a connective tissue. The primary role of Vitamin C is to help this connective tissue. Because collagen is the defense mechanism against disease and infection, and because Vitamin C helps build collagen, it makes sense that it is also a remedy for scurvy by contributing to hemoglobin production. It promotes the production of red blood cells in the bone marrow. Ascorbic acid also supports healthy capillaries, gums, teeth, and even helps heal wounds, burns, and broken tissues. It contributes to hemoglobin and red blood cell production in bone marrow while even preventing blood clots. Another large benefit of this vitamin is the fact that it plays a large role in the production of antibodies. It also functions as a promoter of interferon, a compound that fights cancer.

Found In: Fruits, Grapefruit, Guava, Lemons, Mangos, Orange Juice, Tomatoes, Strawberries, Vegetables, Black Currants, Broccoli, Oranges, Brussels Sprouts, Cabbage, Peppers-Sweet and Hot, Collards, Potatoes, Green Peppers, Kale, Papayas, Rose Hips, Spinach, Tangerines, Watercress.

Calcium: Is the mineral most likely to be deficient in the average diet. Calcium deficiency is a condition in which we fail to receive or to metabolize an adequate supply of calcium. Calcium salts make up about 70% of bone by weight and give your bones its strength and rigidity. Calcium is the chief supportive element in bones and teeth and inadequate levels can lead to osteoporosis.

Iron: Has had therapeutic uses for thousands of years. It was used by the Egyptians to cure baldness and by the Greeks. It was used in wine to restore male potency. It is the most plentiful element on earth and it is an essential trace mineral for humans. Iron is an essential component of hemoglobin, myoglobin and a cofactor of several essential enzymes. Prevents and treats iron-deficiency anemia due to dietary iron deficiency or other causes, stimulates bone marrow production of hemoglobin.

Health Benefits: Essential for protein metabolism, assists in the production of thyroid hormones, connective tissue and several brain neurotransmitters. Maintains a healthy immune system. May help alleviate menstrual pain, may stimulate immunity in iron-deficient people. May promote learning in children with iron deficiency.

Found In: Bread, Egg Yolk, Fish, Red Meats, Garbanzo Beans (chickpeas), Seaweed, Greens, Whole-Grain, Lentils, Liver, Molasses (black strap), Dried Fruits, Poultry, Enriched Cereals, Soybean Flour, Flour.

<u>**Vitamin D**</u>*:* Otherwise known as the sunshine vitamin, is significant in normal body growth and development. In particular, Vitamin D is used to absorb calcium and phosphorus to create bone. Great sources of this supplement include fortified milk, oily fish, liver, and eggs.

Health Benefits: Absorbs calcium and phosphorus to aid in the development of bones and teeth, promotes normal cell growth and maturation. Prevents rickets, maintains a healthy nervous and immune system.

Found In: Cod Liver Oil, Egg Substitutes, Halibut-Liver Oil, Herring, Mackerel, Salmon, Sardines, Sunlight,

<u>**Vitamin E**</u>*:* Otherwise known as alpha-tocopherol, serves as a cofactor in several enzyme systems. It keeps excessive oxidation from occurring that could cause harmful effects in the body. Great sources of Vitamin E may be found in wheat germ, nuts and seeds, whole grain cereals, eggs, and leafy greens.

Health Benefits: Protects fats, cell membranes, DNA, and enzymes against damage, encourages normal growth and development, helps prevent Vitamin E deficiency in premature infants and those with low birth weights. Acts as an antioxidant to protect against heart disease and cancer, anti-blood clotting agent, helps protect against prostate cancer, improves immune system, reduces risk of first fatal heart attack in men.

Found In: Almonds, Asparagus, Avocados, Brazil Nuts, Broc-coli, Canola Oil, Corn, Coconut Oil, Fortified Cereals, Hazelnuts (filberts), Peanuts /Peanut Oil, Safflower Nuts/Oil, Soybean Oil, Spinach, Sunflower Seeds, Walnuts, Wheat Germ, Wheat Germ Oil.

Vitamin K: Otherwise known as phytonadione, promotes production factors critical to normal blood clotting. When foods are processed or cooked, very little of Vitamin K contained in foods is lost. Great sources of this vitamin include dark leafy greens, oils from green plants, and some dairy products.

Health Benefits: Regulates normal blood clotting, promotes normal growth and development essential for kidney functioning.

Found In: Alfalfa, Asparagus, Broccoli, Brussel Sprouts, Cabbage, Greens, Leafy lettuce, Liver, Seaweed, Spinach, Turnip Greens.

Thiamin Vitamin B-1: Is necessary for almost every cellular reaction in the body as a participant in an enzyme system known as thiamin pyrophosphate. It is vital to normal functioning of the nervous system and metabolism. It can be found in meat, whole grains, fish, and nuts.

Benefits: Maintains health of mucous membranes, keeps normal workings of nervous system, heart, and muscles. Helps treat herpes zoster and beriberi, supports normal growth and development, restores deficiencies caused by alcoholism, cirrhosis, overactive thyroid, infection, breast feeding, absorption diseases, pregnancy, prolonged diarrhea, and burns.

Found In: Baked Potato, Beef Kidney/Liver, Brewer's Yeast, Flour; Rye and Whole Grain, Garbanzo Beans, (chickpeas), Dried Kidney Beans, Dried Navy Beans, Orange Juice, Oranges, Peanuts, Peas, Raisins, Brown Rice, and Raw Wheat Germ, Whole-Grain Products.

Riboflavin/Vitamin B-2: Otherwise known as riboflavin, is readily absorbed from foods, such as meat, dairy products, and fortified grains. This vitamin is essential to energy generation, nerve development, blood cell development, and the regulation of certain hormones, releasing food energy for normal growth and development.

Health Benefits: Healthy mucous membrane linings, together with Vitamin A, keeps healthy brain and nervous system, skin, hair, and blood cells.

Found In: Beef, Beef Liver, Organic Dairy Products, Eggs,

Flounder, Herring, Liverwurst, Mackerel, Sardines, Snapper.

Niacin Vitamin B-3: Otherwise known as niacin, acts like other B vitamins to create enzymes that are essential to metabolic cell activity, synthesize hormones, repair genetic material, and maintain normal functioning of the nervous system. Great sources of this vitamin may be found in meat, fish, and whole grains.

Health Benefits: May treat pellagra, decreases cholesterol and triglycerides in blood. Large doses dilate blood vessels, handles ear ringing and dizziness, essential for genetic material repair, potential reduction in heart attacks, depression, and migraine headaches; poor digestion could be improved.

Found In: Beef Liver, Brewer's Yeast, Chicken (white meat), Dried Beans/Peas, Fortified Cereals, Halibut, Peanut Butter, Peanuts, Potatoes, Salmon, Soybeans, Turkey.

Vitamin B6: Otherwise known as pyridoxine, performs as a coenzyme to carry out metabolic processes that affect the body's use of protein, carbohydrates, and fats. It helps to convert tryptophan to niacin, and may be found in meat, fish, eggs, and whole grain foods.

Health Benefits: Promotes healthy cardiovascular, nervous, and immune systems. Supports healthy skin, hair, and normal red blood cell formation, assists in production of food energy, possible anemia treatment, keeps normal homocysteine levels, functions as a tranquilizer, important for healthy nerve and muscle functioning.

Found In: Avocados, Bananas, Beef Liver, Chicken, Fortified Cereals, Ground Beef, Hazelnuts (filberts), Lentils, Potatoes, Salmon, Soybeans, Sunflower Seeds, Wheat germ.

Folate Vitamin B-9: Otherwise known as folic acid, serves as a coenzyme during the creation of DNA. This vitamin is also very important to the growth and reproduction of all body cells, including red blood cells.

Health Benefits: Formation of red blood cells, creation of genetic material, promotes a healthy pregnancy by regulating the nervous system development of the fetus, helps treat anemic patients resulting from folic acid deficiency, functions to metabolize proteins.

***Found In*:** Asparagus, Avocados, Bananas, Beans, Beets, Brewer's Yeast, Brussel Sprouts, Cabbage, Calve's Liver, Cantaloupe, Citrus Fruits/Juices, Endive, Fortified Grain Products, Garbanzo Beans, Green, Leafy Vegetables, Lentils, Sprouts, Wheat Germ.

Vitamin B12*:* Otherwise known as cyanocobalamin, performs as a coenzyme for the creation of DNA material. It also promotes growth and cell development and is important to fat, carbohydrate, and protein metabolism. Although vitamin B-12 is not found in plant foods, good sources of this supplement include meats, fish, eggs, and organic dairy products.

***Health Benefits*:** Growth and development of nerve, skin, hair, and blood cells, helps treat Alzheimer's disease.

***Found In*:** Beef, Beef Liver, Organic Dairy Products, Eggs, Flounder, Herring, Liverwurst, Mackerel, Sardines, Snapper.

Biotin Vitamin H: Is essential to normal growth and development and overall health. Bacteria in the intestines produces enough biotin for the body so that most people would not need an additional supplement of Vitamin H. However, additional great sources of Vitamin H are found in egg yolks, fish, nuts, oatmeal, and beans.

***Health Benefits*:** Essential for release of food energy, reduces symptoms of zinc deficiency, functions in protein metabolism, helps in the formation of fatty acids, could relieve muscle pain and depression.

***Found In*:** Almonds, Bananas, Brewer's Yeast, Brown Rice, Bulgur Wheat, Butter, Calve's Liver, Cashew Nuts, Organic Dairy Products, Cheese, Chicken, Clams, Eggs, Cooked Green Peas, Lentils, Liver, Mackerel, Meats, Mushrooms, Oat Bran, Oatmeal, Peanut Butter Peanuts, Salmon, Soybeans, Split Peas, Walnuts.

Pantothenic Acid Vitamin B-5: Is a coenzyme involved in energy metabolism of carbohydrates, protein, and fat.

***Health Benefits*:** Helps normal growth and development, helps release food energy.

***Found In*:** Avocados, Bananas, Broccoli, Chicken, Collard Greens, Eggs, Lentils, Liver, Meats, Oranges, Peanut Butter, Peanuts, Peas, Soybeans, Sunflower Seeds, Wheat Germ, Whole-Grain Products.

Vitamin P: Otherwise known as flavinoids, enhances the use of Vitamin C by improving absorption and protecting it from oxidation. Great sources of this vitamin are found in the edible pulp of fruits, green pepper, broccoli, and red wine.

Health Benefits: Promotes blood vessel health, including improving capillary strength, prevents accumulation of atherosclerotic plaque. Has anti-inflammatory properties acting against histamines, may help protect against infection and blood vessel disease. May lower blood pressure by relaxing smooth muscle of cardiovascular system. May inhibit tumor growth, may have estrogen-like activity, may prevent hemorrhoids, miscarriages, capillary fragility, nosebleed, retinal bleeding in people with diabetes and hypertension, may lower cholesterol levels.

Found In: Apricots, Blueberry, Black Currants, Broccoli, Buckwheat, Cherries, Citrus Fruits, Ginkgo, Grapes, Green Pepper, Green Tea, Hawthorn, Milk Thistle, Onions, Red Wine, Rose Hips, Tomatoes.

Phosphorus: Is required by the body for bone and teeth formation. Calcium alone can't build strong bones and tissues. New research shows calcium needs phosphorus to maximize its bone-strengthening benefits, and taking a lot of calcium supplements without enough phosphorus could be a waste of money. Phosphorus allows proper digestion of riboflavin and niacin, aids in transmission of nerve impulses, helps your kidneys effectively excrete wastes, gives you stable and plentiful energy, forms the proteins that aid in reproduction, and may help block cancer. Researchers say it's the first time the two elements have been shown to be co-dependent for bone health. Both calcium and phosphorus are found naturally in almonds. More than half of all bone is made from phosphate, and small amounts are also used in the body to maintain tissues and fluids. Taking large amounts of calcium from supplements can interfere with phosphorus absorption.

Iodine: Is a chemical element (as are oxygen, hydrogen, and iron). Iodine comes in three commercial forms, calcium iodide, potassium iodide, and sodium iodide. Iodine affects the human body in many ways. It is known to be essential in maintaining the function of the thyroid and parathyroid glands in the human body. It is also essential to the production of thyroxine, a hormone associated with the thyroid gland and proper thyroid functioning. The thyroid is a butterfly-shaped gland in the front part of the neck. It makes two hormones (thyroxine (T4) and tri-iodothyronine (T3)). The thyroid hormones are released into the bloodstream and carried by it to target organs, particularly the liver, kidneys, muscles, heart, and the developing brain. Iodine also promotes general growth and development within the body as well as aiding in metabolism. Iodine, because of its role in metabolism, also helps to burn off excess fat. Celtic Sea Salt is the best source of naturally-balanced iodine.

Magnesium: Is one of the most plentiful minerals in the soft tissue. It is found in high concentrations inside cells, namely those of the brain and heart. The average adult body contains around 20-28g of magnesium with about 60% of it present in the bones. The rest is in the muscle, soft tissue and body fluids.

Health Benefits: Assists bone growth, aids function of nerves and muscles, including regulation of normal heart rhythm, conducts nerve impulses. Works as a laxative in large doses, acts as antacid in small doses. Strengthens tooth enamel, produces and transfers energy in the body, maintains healthy heart, bones, muscles and blood vessels. Important in protein and carbohydrate metabolism, aids in the transport of substances across cell membranes.

Found In: Almonds, Herring, Avocados, Leafy Green Vegetables, Bananas, Mackerel, Bluefish, Molasses, Carp, Nuts, Cod, Ocean Perch, Collards, Beet Greens, Organic Dairy Products, Flounder, Wheat Germ, Whole Wheat Bread, Peanuts, Baked Beans, Beet Greens, Brown Rice, cooked; Kidney Beans, Cashew Nuts, Spinach, Chick Peas, Black-Eyed Peas, Artichokes, Apricots, Sweet Corn, Green Peas, Raisins, Whole-Wheat Spaghetti, Avocado, Oatmeal.

Potassium: Is found in several different forms, including Potassium Chloride, the most common form. It has many functions in the body such as playing a role in protein synthesis and for the conversion of blood sugar in to glycogen (sugar). It triggers a number of enzymes, namely those concerned with energy production. The average human body contains about 140g of potassium.

Health Benefits: Promotes regular heartbeat, normal muscle contraction, regulates transfer of nutrients to cells, maintains water balance in body tissues and cells, restores normal function of nerve cells, heart cells, skeletal muscle cells, kidneys, stomach-juice secretion. An enzyme (adenosine triphosphatase) controls the flow of potassium and sodium into and out of cells to maintain normal function of the heart, brain, skeletal muscles and kidney, and to maintain acid-base balance.

Found In: Fruits, Vegetables Whole Grains, Asparagus, Molasses, Avocados, Nuts, Bananas, Parsnips, Beans, Peas (fresh), Cantaloupe, Potatoes, Carrots, Raisins, Chard, Citrus Fruit, Sardines, Spinach, fresh and boiled; Snapper, grilled; Prunes, Pistachios, Peanuts, Melon, Green Peas, boiled; Barley, Beef.

Zinc: Is an essential mineral that is found in every cell in our body. It stimulates the activity of about 100 enzymes, substances that promote biochemical reactions in your body. Among its many functions, zinc helps maintain a healthy immune system, is needed for wound healing, helps maintain your sense of taste and smell, and is needed for DNA synthesis. Taking lozenges made of zinc gluconate can help shorten the length of a cold.. Take 15 mg of zinc daily (the amount in most multivitamins). Because zinc can block copper absorption, make sure that your supplement also contains 1 to 2 mg of copper. Consuming zinc on an empty stomach can cause nausea, so take zinc supplements with food.

Selenium: Could be your most potent ally against cancer. Selenium is a trace element found naturally in foods like nuts and liver. Nearly all of the selenium in animal tissue is found in the proteins. Some of these proteins contain stoichiometric quantities of selenium and are known as selenoproteins. Other proteins contain variable amounts of selenium (which substitute sulfur randomly in the original protein) and are known as selenium-binding proteins. Researchers for more than 20 years of animal studies have suggested that tiny amounts of selenium in the diet can reduce the risk of cancer in several organs, but much less is known about the anti-cancer benefits of selenium in humans. In recent years, laboratory experiments, clinical trials and epidemiological data have established the role of selenium in the prevention of a number of degenerative conditions including cancer, inflammatory diseases, cardiovascular diseases, neurological diseases, aging, and infections. Most of these effects are related to the function of selenium in the antioxidant enzyme systems. A study at the University of Arizona in Tucson in 1996 found that people who took 200 mcg of selenium a day for four and a half years reduced their risk of cancer by 32% and their risk of death from cancer by 50%. Celtic Sea Salt is the best source of this vitally important mineral. Numerous research reports indicate that higher blood levels of selenium lowers mortality from cancer including lung, colorectal, prostate and skin cancer.

Laboratory studies indicate the potentially beneficial role of selenium in the management of mammary cancer. Selenium is an antioxidant and appears to regenerate Vitamins E and C so that they can continue to fight free radicals. Be aware that doses of more than 400 mcg daily can be toxic. Research also shows that a lower anti-oxidant status has been linked to higher incidence of cardiovascular diseases due to increased levels of LDL oxidation. Selenium is one of the antioxidants that may help to inhibit LDL oxidation. Low selenium status has been associated with the incidence of arthritis. Studies show the beneficial role of selenium as a free radical that delays the progression of this condition. Low levels of selenium in HIV /AIDS sufferers have been linked to higher mortality. Low plasma selenium status has also been linked with senility and cognitive decline in the elderly and with Alzheimer's disease, antioxidant enzymes leading to a number of functional disorders including skeletal muscle dysfunction, cardiac dysfunction, hepatic degradation.

Copper: Is essential for life, which means that the human body must have copper to stay healthy. This mineral helps transport oxygen through your body, maintain hair color, and is used to make hormones. In fact, for a variety of biochemical processes in the body to operate normally, copper must be a part of our diet. To be healthy, you need a diet adequate in protein, carbohydrates, fats, vitamins, and minerals. Essential trace minerals, including copper, are needed only in very small amounts, which is why they are called micro-nutrients.

Health Benefits: Copper stimulates the immune system to fight infections, repair injured tissues, and promote healing. Copper also helps to neutralize "free-radicals" which can cause severe damage to cells. Copper is also needed for certain critical enzymes to function in the body.

Found In: Vegetables (potatoes), Legumes (beans and peas), Nuts (peanuts and pecans), Grains (wheat and rye), Fruits (peach and raisin), and, yes, even Chocolate.

<u>Manganese:</u> Is a mineral element that is nutritionally essential. The derivation of its name from the Greek word for magic remains appropriate, because scientists are still working to understand the diverse effects of manganese deficiency. Manganese is an antioxidant nutrient that is important in the breakdown of amino acids and the production of energy. It is necessary for the metabolism of Vitamin B-1 and Vitamin E and it activates various enzymes which are important for proper digestion and utilization of foods. Manganese is a catalyst in the breakdown of fats and cholesterol. It helps nourish the nerves and brain, is necessary for normal skeletal development, and helps to maintain sex hormone production and to regulate blood sugar levels.

<u>Chromium:</u> This mineral helps the hormone insulin work more efficiently, making it an especially important nutrient for people who have Type II Diabetes or are at risk for developing it. Insulin usually helps lower blood sugar levels, but if you have Type II Diabetes, your insulin is less effective. In fact, some cases of Type II diabetes are actually triggered by a chromium deficiency. Chromium's effect on insulin may also help you lose weight. Studies show that it can help you hold on to muscle while shedding fat.

Health Benefits: Chromium has been used for diabetes, high cholesterol and low blood sugar (hypoglycemia) and is backed by a great deal of scientific research. Chromium has also been used for weight loss, to increase athletic performance and depression.

Found In: Liver, Wheat Germ, Many meats, Fish, Fruits, Whole Grains, and Vegetables, Carrots, Potatoes, Spinach, Alfalfa, Brown Sugar (raw), Molasses.

<u>Chloride:</u> Is one of the most important minerals in the blood, along with sodium, potassium, and calcium. Chloride helps keep the amount of fluid inside and outside of cells in balance. It also helps maintain proper blood volume, blood pressure, and pH of body fluids. Chloride is a binary compound of chlorine; a salt of hydrochloric

acid. Chloride ions are secreted in the gastric juice as hydrochloric acid, which is essential for the digestion of food. Chloride is the major extracellular anion and contributes to many body functions including the maintenance of osmotic pressure, acid-base balance, muscular activity, and the movement of water between fluid compartments. Chloride is absorbed by the intestine during food digestion. Any excess chloride is passed out of the body through the urine. Chloride levels in the blood generally rise and fall along with sodium levels in the blood. The amount of chloride in the blood is indirectly regulated by the hormone aldosterone, which also regulates the amount of sodium in the blood. **Remember, God has placed before you life and death, sickness and disease, so choose life, that you and your seed may live.**

CHAPTER 17

The 28 Day Health Challenge

Healing • Weight Loss • Cleansing • Detox

No amount of medications, diet pills, or by-pass surgery, no matter how much they cost can promote total internal and external body healing, weight loss, cleansing and detoxing. Remember, just because you may not be overweight on the outside, your internal organs like your heart, liver, and kidneys, can be covered in excess fatty tissue. This internal condition is just as hazardous as external obesity. Your internal organs cannot function properly if they are saturated with fat.

If you suffer from any of the following conditions: Cancer, Diabetes, Heart Disease, Hypertension, Obesity, Arthritis, Osteoporosis, Eczema, AIDS, MS, Alzheimer's Disease, Fibromyalgia, High Cholesterol, Malnutrition, Muscle Cramps, Kidney Stones, Gallstones, Gout, Indigestion, Chronic Fatigue Syndrome, Lupus, Hiatal Hernia, Heartburn, High Blood Pressure, Premature Aging and Greying, Acne, Menopause, PMS Complications, Skin Rashes, Insomnia, Anemia, Irritable Bowel Syndrome, and many, many more, take the 28-day challenge to reverse and begin the healing process from all the above mentioned afflictions. God has allowed you to defile the temple for many years as a living sacrifice. The least you can do is offer back to Him just 28 days. It is time to reverse the transfer of your health and wealth back into the Kingdom of God.

For the next 28 days, do the following:

1) Start each morning out with **prayer** and your favorite **worship songs**. This means that you may have to go to bed 15 to 20 minutes earlier than normal so you can get up a little earlier.

2) **Read** your **Bible** for at least 30 minutes a day, and study certain passages of scripture as you are led by the Spirit.

3) Total body ultimate cleanse by Nature's Secret or Para Cleanse.

4) Use only first cold press, extra virgin olive oil or Smart Balance

buttery spread in place of all oils.

5)   Use Celtic Sea Salt in place of table salt and all seasonings salts.

6)   Use stevia (diabetic friendly), honey, or 100% pure maple syrup in place of all sweeteners.

7)   Drink only distilled water; add grapefruit seed extract 1-2 times daily.

8)   Take 2 Tbsp of organic flaxseed oil w/ligans(shake well), 2 Tbsp extra virgin olive oil sprinkled with Celtic Salt daily.

9)   Take one clove of organic garlic twice daily chopped up and place into a gel-cap.

10)   Think positive thoughts and try to read something that makes you   laugh. Also, don't hang out with argumentative people and those who seem to always be depressed.

In severe cases additional cleansing may be necessary. If so email sales@blessandeat.com

Day 1: Fast with distilled water and juice all day. If you don't have a juicer, a blender is okay. Blend together 2 to 3 apples, 2 sticks of celery, 1/8 tsp Celtic Sea Salt, and 1/4 cup of distilled water. Drink this once every 4 hours. In between juicing, drink 3 glasses of distilled water mixed with fresh-squeezed lemon juice, and 3 or 4 shakes of Celtic Sea Salt. This is the most important day, so it is necessary that you try to follow these directions closely. Remember, Celtic Sea Salt is naturally balanced with more than 85 minerals and trace minerals, which actually helps to balance and regulate all bodily functions including blood pressure, heart function and blood sugar levels.
Days 2-7: Drink 20-24oz. of warm distilled water first thing in the morning in addition to the following:

Breakfast: Have fruits like melons, apples, grapefruits, pears, oranges, grapes, etc. Blend into a fruit drink if you like, add a pinch of Celtic Sea Salt and celery. All fruits should be organic whenever possible.

Lunch: Have a salad with mixed greens, sprinkled with almonds, sunflower seeds, ground flax seed, pumpkin seeds, cucumbers, tomatoes, and any other type of vegetables. Use an organic salad dressing only or make your own. No fruit with this meal. Snack on fruit between meals. Children can eat a vegetable sandwich.

Dinner: Covenant Salad(bottom of page) can be served over a bed of organic spring mix salad or fresh organic spinach.

Day 8: Same as Day 1.

Days 9-14: Same as Days 2-7

Day 15: Same as Day 1.

Days 16-21: Same as Days 2-7.

Day 22: Same as Day 1.

Days 23-28: Same as Days 2-7.

For the next 28 days avoid all of the following:

1.   All meats, chicken, seafood and fish.

2.   All fried, baked (except organic whole seven-grain bread, Daniel's bread, or homemade wheat bread) and processed foods.

3.   All dairy and dairy products to include milk, cheese, yogurt, ice cream, sour cream, etc. All eggs and products containing eggs.

4.   All margarine, buttery spreads, and cooking oils like Crisco, Mazola, etc.

5.   All refined sugar, table salt, artificial sweeteners, syrups, and seasoning salts.

6.   All processed and bleached wheat products, white rice, pasta.

7.   All soft drinks, diet sodas, fruit juices, coffee, and products containing caffeine. All alcohol and tobacco products.

Covenant Salad: (The Healing Salad) 1 chopped Cucumber, Tomato, Avocado, 1 bag of frozen green peas, string beans, ½ bag sweet corn, fresh garlic,1 cup chopped broccoli, ½ cup ground flaxseed, 5 Tbsp. extra virgin olive oil, 4 Tbsp flax seed oil, ½ cup chopped onions, black pepper, Celtic Sea salt, non-irradiated herbal seasoning, fresh-squeezed lemon juice, sesame seeds, raw almonds, pumpkin seeds and cilantro. Mix all of these ingredients together in a large bowl and season to taste. Hanover brand vegetables are okay if organic vegetables are not available. This salad packs quite a healthy punch. It contains heart healthy Omega 3, 6, and 9 essential fatty oils, vitamins and over 80 minerals and trace minerals, antioxidants, phytochemical nutrients, dietary fiber, potassium, iron, magnesium, Vitamin B1, Vitamin B2, Vitamin B6, niacin, phosphorous, Vitamin C, Vitamin A, calcium, and many, many more. Covenant Salad contains the nutrients and minerals needed to assist the body in healing itself of degenerative diseases like heart disease and cancer, arthritis, skin conditions, diabetes, diminished immune function and premenstrual syndrome, decreased memory and mental abilities, tingling sensation of the nerves, poor vision, increased tendency to form blood clots, increased triglycerides and "bad" cholesterol levels, impaired membrane function, hypertension, irregular heart beat, learning disorders, and menopausal discomfort. **Remember, God has placed before you life and death, sickness and disease, so choose life, that you and your seed may live.**

For more educational information regarding recipes and nutritious meal preparations, write to:

Bless It & Eat It

P.O. Box 5074

Fredericksburg VA 22406

or send an e-mail to: sales@blessandeat.com

References

Scripture References: NIV Study Bible, Nelson Study Bible, The Reese Chronological Bible, Dakes Annotated Reference Bible.
Additional References: Vines Complete Expository Dictionary, Baxter's Explore The Book, Evangelical Dictionary of Theology, The Strongest Strong's Exhaustive Concordance of the Bible, Lecture in Systematic Theology, Manners Customs Of The Bible, Miracle Food Cures From The Bible, Natural Healing Cures Of the Bible, Prescription for Herbal Healing.
Kohn L, ed, Corrigan J, ed, Donaldson M, ed. To Err Is Human: Building a Safer Health System. Washington, DC: National Academy Press; 1999.
Leape L. Unnecessary surgery. Annu Rev Public Health. 1992;13:368-383
Phillips D, Christenfeld N, Glynn L. Increase in US medication-error deaths between 1983 and 1993.Lancent. 1998;351:643-644.
Lazarou J, Pomeranz B, Corey P. Incidence of adverse drug reactions in JAMA. 1998;279:1200-1205
Arthur JR. The role of selenium in thyroid hormone metabolism. Can J Physiol Pharmacol 1991;69:1648-52.
Hercberg S, Galan P, Preziosi P, Roussel AM, Arnaud J, Richard MJ, Malvy D, Paul-Dauphin A, Briancon S, Favier A. Background and rationale behind the SU.VI.MAX Study, a prevention trial using nutritional doses of a combination of antioxidant vitamins and minerals to reduce cardiovascular diseases and cancers. Supplementation en Vitamines et Mineraux AntiXydants Study. Int J Vitam Nutr Res 1998;68:3-20
Kiremidjian-Schumacher L,. & Roy M.(1998). Selenium and Immune Function. Suppl 1:50-6 Levander OA. Scientific rationale for the 1989 recommended dietary allowance for selenium. J Am Diet Assoc 1991;91:1572-6.
Sources: Blaurock-Busch, E. pH.D. Mineral and Trace Element Analysis. Boulder, CO. TMI/MTM Books. 1996. Jensen, B. DC, pH.D. Come Alive! Total Health through an Understanding of Minerals, Trace Elements & Electrolytes. Escondido, CA. Jensen. 1997.
Bergner, P. The Healing Power of Minerals, Special Nutrients, and Trace Elements. Rocklin, CA. Pima Publishing. 1997. Fallon, S. Nourishing Traditions. Washington D.C. New Trends Publishing.1999 .
David Goldstein, "Up Close: A Beef With Dairy," KCAL, 30 May 02.

"Mad Cow Casts Light on Beef Uses," Los Angeles Times, 4 Jan. 2004.

David R. Winston, "Goals for Heifer Rearing," Department of Dairy Science, Virginia Polytech University, 1 Oct. 1996.

Anne Karpf, "Dairy Monsters," The Guardian, 13 Dec. 2003

Richard L. Wallace, D.V.M., M.S., "Market Cows: A Potential Profit Center," University of Illinois at Urbana-Champaign, 2004.

National Agriculture Statistics Service, "Milk Production," United States Department of Agriculture, 17 Feb. 2004.

Don P. Blaney, The Changing Landscape of U.S. Milk Production, Statistical Bulletin Number 978, United States Department of Agriculture, Jun. 2002.

David Pace, "Feeding a Bucket Calf," Oklahoma Cooperative Extension Service, Oklahoma State University.

"Mad Cow Case Casts Light on Beef Uses," Los Angeles Times, 4 Jan. 2004.

Helen Pearson, "Udder Suicide, E.Coli Kill off Milk-Making Mammary"Cells," Nature, 6 Aug. 2001.

Guidelines on Normal and Abnormal Raw Milk Based on Somatic Cell Counts and Signs of Clinical Mastitis," National Mastitis Council, 2001. P.L. Ruegg, "Practical Food Safety Interventions for Dairy Production," Journal of Dairy Science, 86 (2003):E1-E9.

National Mastitis Council.

S. Waage et al., "Identification of Risk Factors for Clinical Mastitis in Dairy Heifers," Journal of Dairy Science, 81 (1998): 1275-84.

Morten Dam Rasmussen et al., "The Impact of Automatic Milking on Udder Health," Proceedings of the Second International Symposium on Mastitis and Milk Quality, Vancouver, B.C.: 2001. Michael Raine, "Cloning—New Era in Breeding Technology Raises Hopes, Concerns," The Western Producer, 17 Jul. 2002.

Susan C. Kahler, "Raising Contented Cattle Makes Welfare, Production Sense," Journal of the American Veterinary Medical Association, 15 Jan. 2001.

Food Safety and Inspection Service, "Safety of Veal, From Farm to Table," USDA, Feb. 2003.

John M. Smith, "Raising Dairy Veal," Ohio State University, information adapted from the Guide for the Care and Production of Veal Calves, 4th ed., 1993, American Veal Association, Inc.

" The European Food Information Council, 2003.

Marla Cone, "State Dairy Farms Try to Clean Up Their Act," Los Angeles Times, 28 Apr. 1998.

John Heilprin, "Bush Issues Rule for Factory-Style Farms," Associated Press, 16 Dec. 2002.

Marlow Vesterby and Kenneth S. Krupa, "Major Uses of Land in the United States, 1997," Statistical Bulletin Number 973, United States Department of Agriculture, 1997.

Dick Grant, "Water Quality and Requirements for Dairy Cattle," NebGuide, Cooperative Extension, Institute of Agriculture and Natural Resources, University of Nebraska-Lincoln, 1996.

Bill McKibben, "Taking the Pulse of the Planet," Audubon, Nov. 1999: 104.

"Beef Cattle Farming in Ontario," Ontario Farm Animal Council, 12 Feb. 2004.

USDA National Nutrient Database for Standard Reference, "Milk, Whole, 3.25% Milkfat," 16 Jul. 2003.

USDA National Nutrient Database for Standard Reference, "Milk, Human, Mature, Fluid," 16 Jul. 2003.

American Gastroenterological Association, "American Gastroenterolo- gical Association Medical Position Statement: Guidelines for the Evaluation of Food Allergies," Gastroenterology 120 (2001): 1023-5. National Digestive Diseases Information Clearinghouse, "Lactose Intolerance," National Institute of Diabetes and Digestive and Kidney Diseases, Mar. 2003.

Courtney Taylor, "Got Milk (Intolerance)? Digestive Malady Affects 30-50 Million," The Clarion-Ledger, 1 Aug. 2003.

"Milk Protein May Play Role in Mental Disorders," Reuters Health, 1 Apr. 1999.

Severin Carrell, "Milk Causes 'Serious Illness for 7M Britons.' Scientists Say Undetected Lactose Intolerance Is to Blame for Chronic Fatigue, Arthritis and Bowel Problems," The Independent, 22 Jun.

About the Author

Pastor Jonathan Finley is fast becoming the leading voice within the body of Christ regarding the dangers of ignoring the physical person. He has been an advocate in supporting biblical nutritional principals for more than 25 years. His mission has been focused on bringing awareness to the body of Christ in order to prevent and reverse degenerative diseases. He shows how, through the art of deception, the adversary has depleted our physical bodies of vital substances that are required to keep the Temple of the Holy Spirit prospering and in good health. John is actively pursuing every possible resource that will help save as many children and adults as possible from the prospect of having to live with generational degenerative diseases such as cancer, diabetes, heart disease, hypertension, obesity, and a myriad of other common afflictions. John's life passion is to help everyone live in true prosperity, spiritually and physically, the whole person. He believes too many people are needlessly suffering and dying prematurely, and that many of them are not seeking biblical answers to their problems. With so many people now suffering with a myriad of afflictions simultaneously, John believes it is time to uncover the veil of deception that has just as many believers suffering as nonbelievers. Pastor John is available for personal appearances, seminars, and book signings on a limited basis. Call 540-371-0486 or e-mail:
sales @blessandeat.com for more information or go to www.blessandeat.com.

Dedication

This book is dedicated to my mother and father in their loving memory. I thank God for my parents who reared me up to understand that the first sign of wisdom is the fear of God. Although they are no longer with us physically, it is great to know spiritually we are all connected because we worship the same living God. I thank God for my lovely wife of almost 20 years who has stood with me through every test and trial. I love you, Spice, with all my heart. I thank God for my four beautiful children and one grandson who are my inspiration and motivation. I want to give a special thanks to the Virtuous Ministries Family for the love and support that you have given to help support the vision God has given Lynne and I. I deeply thank every prayer intercessor and warrior around the country. Keep on keeping on in the precious name of our Lord and Savior Jesus Christ.